BLACK HALLOWEEN MAKEUP

TABLE OF CONTENTS

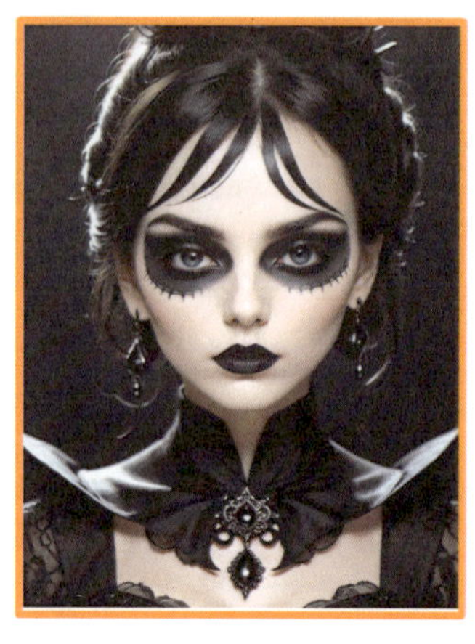
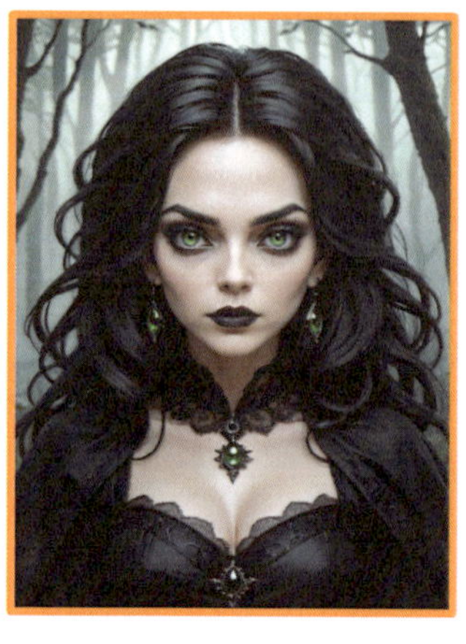
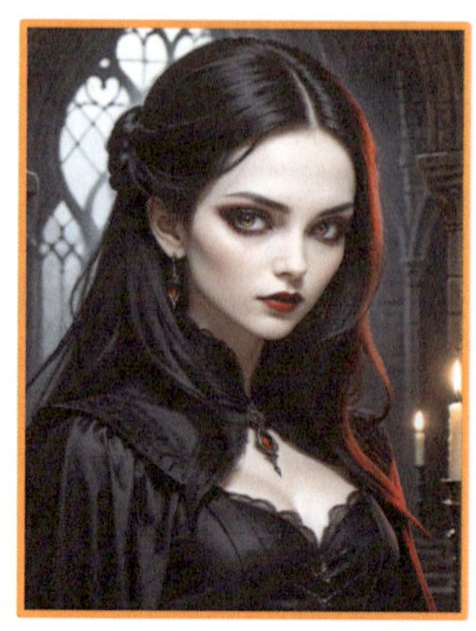
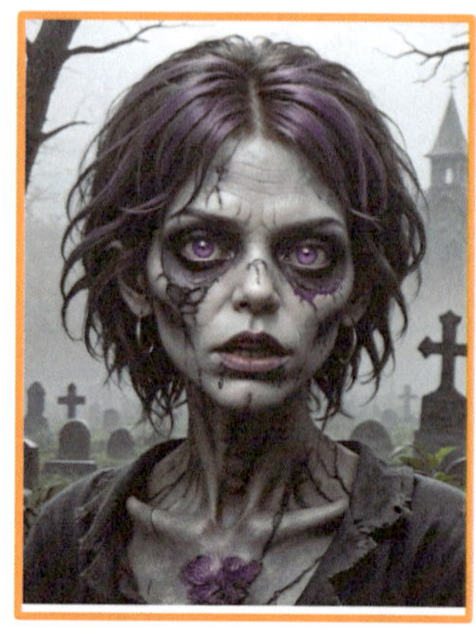
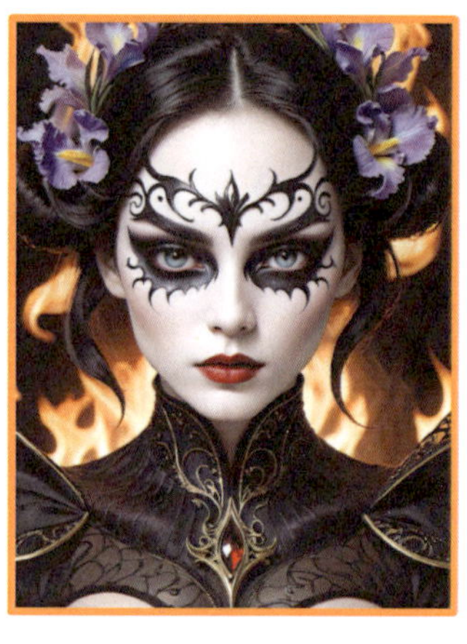
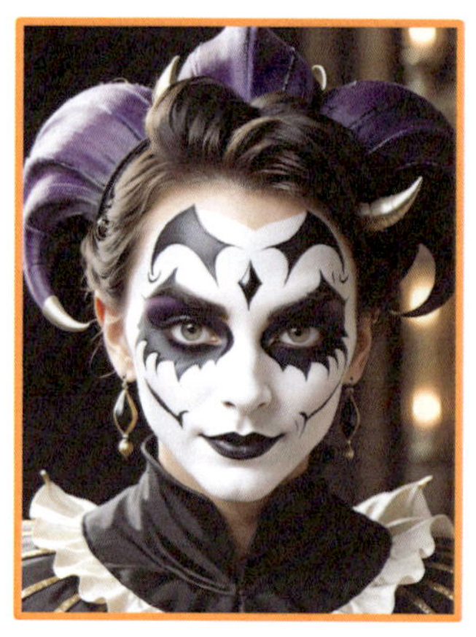
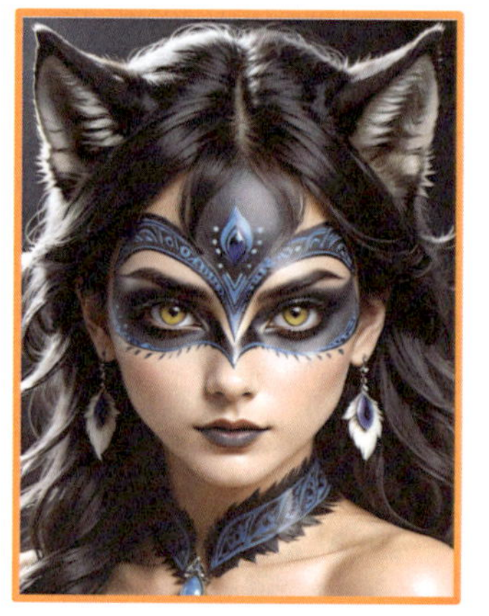
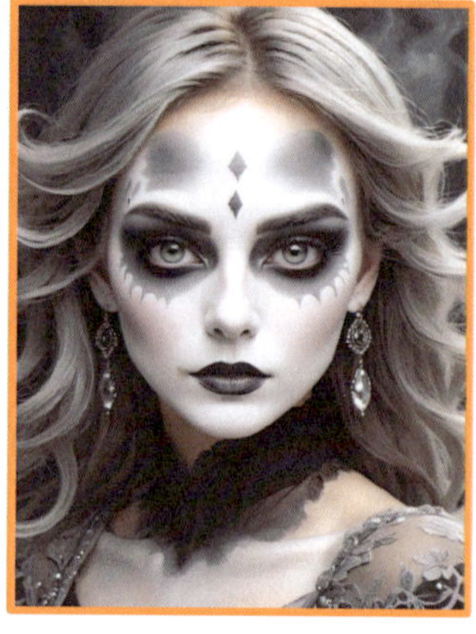
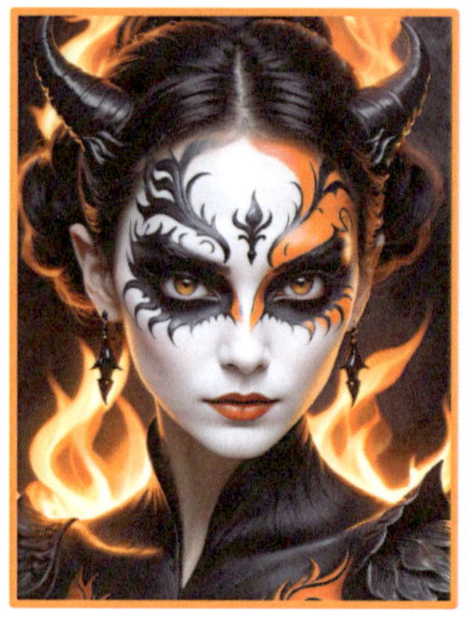
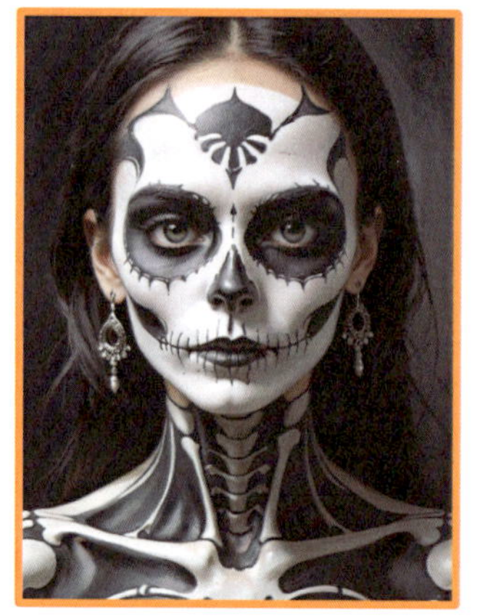
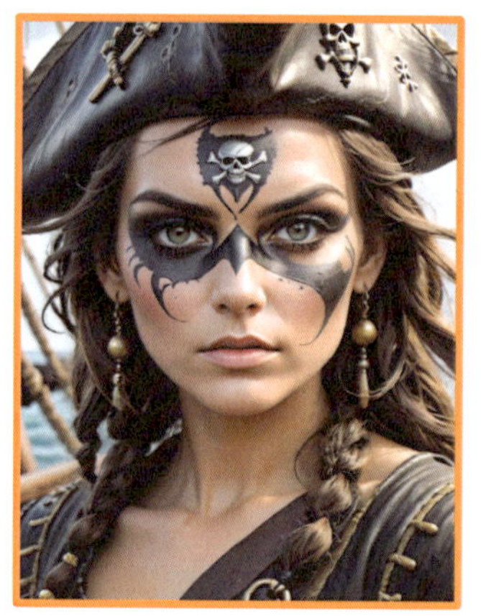
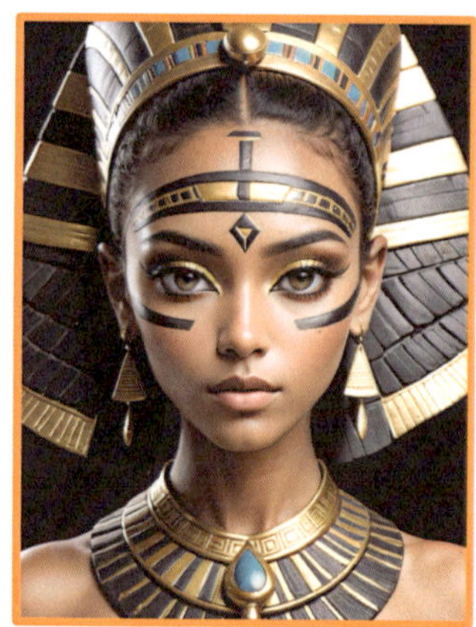
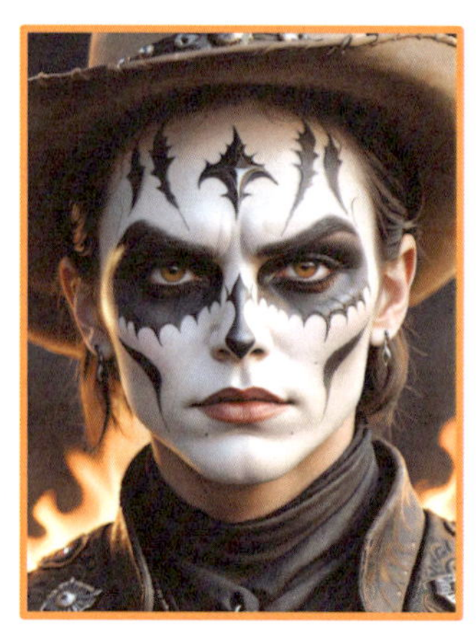
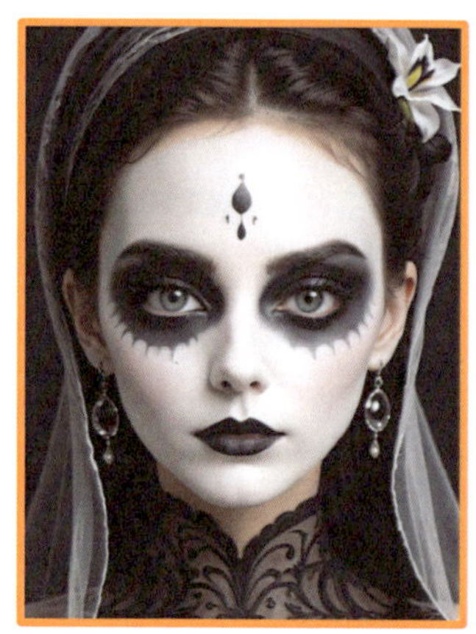
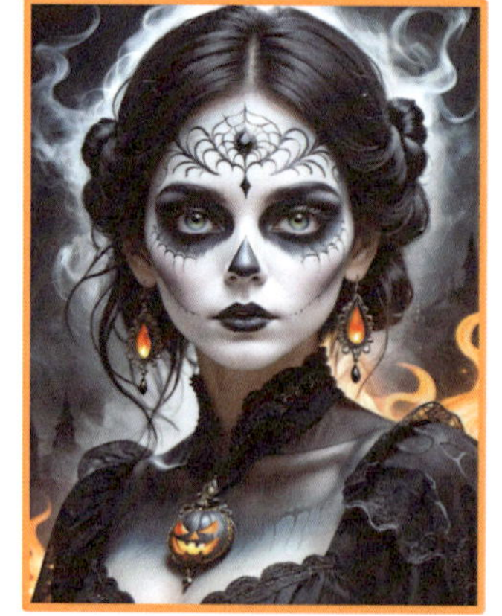
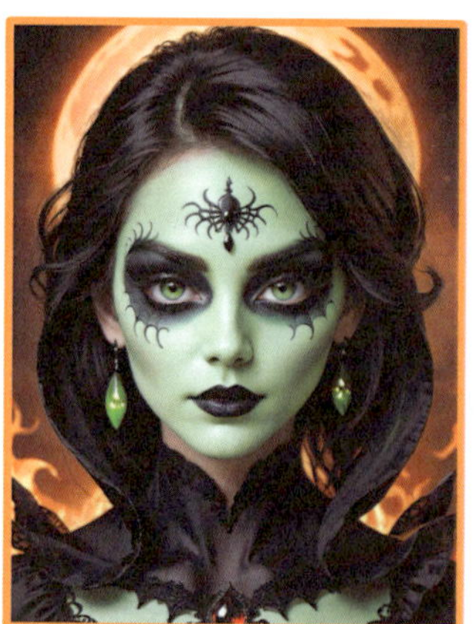

INTRODUCTION TO THE BOOK

WELCOME TO THE WORLD OF HALLOWEEN MAKEUP, WHERE EVERY FACE BECOMES A CANVAS, AND EVERY CREATION TELLS A STORY.

THIS BOOK IS DESIGNED FOR ALL HALLOWEEN ENTHUSIASTS, FROM THOSE JUST BEGINNING THEIR MAKEUP JOURNEY TO THOSE LOOKING TO REFINE THEIR SKILLS. OUR DETAILED STEP-BY-STEP INSTRUCTIONS WILL GUIDE YOU THROUGH THE PROCESS OF CREATING STUNNING, DARK, AND UNIQUE LOOKS THAT WILL CAPTIVATE YOUR FRIENDS AND FAMILY.

EACH STYLE IN THIS BOOK HAS BEEN CRAFTED TO BE BOTH VISUALLY STRIKING AND EASY TO RECREATE. WHETHER YOU WANT TO BECOME A DARK WITCH, A DEVILISH JESTER, OR AN ICY QUEEN, YOU'LL FIND SOMETHING HERE TO INSPIRE YOU. OUR INSPIRATIONS DRAW FROM VARIOUS CULTURES, MYTHS, AND LEGENDS TO CREATE UNFORGETTABLE LOOKS FOR THE SPOOKIEST NIGHT OF THE YEAR.

REMEMBER, MAKEUP IS NOT JUST A WAY TO CHANGE YOUR APPEARANCE — IT'S AN ART FORM THAT ALLOWS YOU TO EXPRESS YOURSELF, STEP INTO ANOTHER ROLE, AND CREATE A ONE-OF-A-KIND ATMOSPHERE. WITH EACH BRUSHSTROKE, WITH EVERY APPLIED COLOR, YOU ARE CREATING SOMETHING EXTRAORDINARY. OUR GUIDES WILL LEAD YOU THROUGH EACH STEP, BUT THE FINAL INTERPRETATION IS YOURS TO MAKE.

DON'T FORGET TO TAKE CARE OF YOUR HEALTH AND SAFETY WHILE CREATING YOUR MAKEUP MASTERPIECES BY FOLLOWING THE BHP (HEALTH AND SAFETY) GUIDELINES PROVIDED BELOW. ENJOY THE CREATIVE PROCESS AND HAVE FUN EXPLORING THE MAGIC OF HALLOWEEN!

HEALTH AND SAFETY GUIDELINES FOR MAKEUP APPLICATION

CLEAN HANDS:

ALWAYS WASH YOUR HANDS BEFORE AND AFTER APPLYING MAKEUP. CLEAN HANDS PREVENT THE TRANSFER OF BACTERIA TO YOUR SKIN AND MAKEUP PRODUCTS, MINIMIZING THE RISK OF INFECTIONS.

TOOL HYGIENE:

ENSURE THAT ALL MAKEUP TOOLS, SUCH AS BRUSHES, SPONGES, AND APPLICATORS, ARE CLEAN BEFORE USE. REGULARLY WASH YOUR BRUSHES AND REPLACE SPONGES TO AVOID THE BUILDUP OF BACTERIA AND COSMETIC RESIDUE.

PRODUCT TESTING:

BEFORE APPLYING NEW COSMETICS TO YOUR FACE, CONDUCT AN ALLERGY TEST. APPLY A SMALL AMOUNT OF THE PRODUCT ON THE INSIDE OF YOUR WRIST OR BEHIND YOUR EAR AND WAIT 24 HOURS TO ENSURE IT DOESN'T CAUSE AN ALLERGIC REACTION.

AVOID CONTACT WITH EYES:

WHEN APPLYING COSMETICS AROUND THE EYES, BE ESPECIALLY CAREFUL. AVOID GETTING MAKEUP INTO YOUR EYES TO PREVENT IRRITATION OR DAMAGE.

SAFE STORAGE OF COSMETICS:

STORE COSMETICS IN A COOL, DRY PLACE AWAY FROM DIRECT SUNLIGHT. ENSURE THEY ARE TIGHTLY SEALED TO AVOID CONTAMINATION AND EXTEND THEIR SHELF LIFE.

EXPIRATION DATES:

PAY ATTENTION TO THE EXPIRATION DATES OF COSMETICS. DO NOT USE PRODUCTS BEYOND THEIR EXPIRATION DATE, AS THEY MAY LOSE THEIR EFFECTIVENESS OR BECOME UNSAFE FOR YOUR SKIN.

SKIN REST:

AFTER THE EVENT OR PHOTO SESSION, REMEMBER TO THOROUGHLY CLEANSE YOUR FACE OF ALL MAKEUP PRODUCTS. ALLOW YOUR SKIN TO BREATHE AND REJUVENATE BY APPLYING A MOISTURIZING CREAM.

AVOID SHARING COSMETICS:

MAKEUP PRODUCTS SUCH AS LIPSTICKS, MASCARAS, AND FOUNDATIONS ARE MEANT FOR PERSONAL USE. SHARING THEM CAN LEAD TO THE SPREAD OF BACTERIA AND VIRUSES.

USE SAFE PRODUCTS:

MAKE SURE ALL THE COSMETICS YOU USE ARE SAFE FOR SKIN APPLICATION AND HAVE THE APPROPRIATE SAFETY CERTIFICATIONS. AVOID PRODUCTS CONTAINING INGREDIENTS TO WHICH YOU ARE ALLERGIC.

FOLLOWING THESE HEALTH AND SAFETY GUIDELINES WILL HELP YOU ENJOY CREATING MAKEUP LOOKS IN A SAFE AND HYGIENIC MANNER, ENSURING THE BEST RESULTS WITHOUT COMPROMISING YOUR HEALTH. CREATE, EXPERIMENT, AND HAVE FUN, ALL WHILE STAYING SAFE!

BLACK WIDOW"

STEP-BY-STEP INSTRUCTIONS:

1. SKIN PREPARATION:

TOOLS: LIGHT FOUNDATION, TRANSLUCENT POWDER.

INSTRUCTIONS: APPLY LIGHT FOUNDATION ALL OVER THE FACE TO ACHIEVE A SMOOTH, EVEN COMPLEXION. ENSURE THE FOUNDATION IS EVENLY BLENDED, CREATING A PERFECT BASE FOR THE INTENSE, BLACK MAKEUP.

2. EYES:

TOOLS: BLACK EYESHADOW, BLACK EYELINER, MASCARA, BLACK CONTACT LENSES (OPTIONAL).

INSTRUCTIONS: APPLY BLACK EYESHADOW ON THE UPPER AND LOWER LIDS, BLENDING IT TOWARDS THE BROWS AND TEMPLES TO CREATE A DEEP, GOTHIC EFFECT. USE BLACK EYELINER TO DRAW BOLD LINES AROUND THE EYES, EXTENDING THEM TOWARDS THE OUTER CORNERS. APPLY MASCARA TO ADD VOLUME AND LENGTH TO THE LASHES. FOR AN EVEN MORE DRAMATIC EFFECT, CONSIDER WEARING BLACK CONTACT LENSES.

3. EYEBROWS:

TOOLS: BLACK FACE PAINT OR EYELINER.

INSTRUCTIONS: DEFINE THE EYEBROWS, GIVING THEM A SHARP, DRAMATIC SHAPE THAT ENHANCES THE INTENSITY OF THE EYE MAKEUP. THE EYEBROWS SHOULD BE WELL-DEFINED TO ADD A MYSTERIOUS TOUCH TO THE GAZE.

4. LIPS:

TOOLS: BLACK LIPSTICK.

INSTRUCTIONS: APPLY INTENSE BLACK LIPSTICK, CAREFULLY OUTLINING THE LIPS. THE LIPS SHOULD LOOK BOLD AND DRAMATIC, COMPLEMENTING THE DARK EYE MAKEUP.

5. DETAILS:

TOOLS: BLACK FACE PAINT, FINE BRUSH.

INSTRUCTIONS: USE BLACK FACE PAINT TO ADD DELICATE, STYLIZED LINES AND PATTERNS ON THE FOREHEAD, RESEMBLING SPIDER LEGS, SYMBOLIZING THE BLACK WIDOW. THE PATTERNS SHOULD BE PRECISE AND SYMMETRICAL.

6. FINISHING TOUCHES:

TOOLS: BLACK WIG OR HAIR STYLED BLACK, ELEGANT GOTHIC JEWELRY, BLACK DRESS.

INSTRUCTIONS: COMPLETE THE LOOK BY WEARING A BLACK WIG OR STYLING THE HAIR IN BLACK. ADD ELEGANT GOTHIC JEWELRY, SUCH AS EARRINGS AND A NECKLACE WITH BLACK STONES. FINALLY, WEAR A BLACK DRESS TO COMPLETE THE GOTHIC, DARK APPEARANCE.

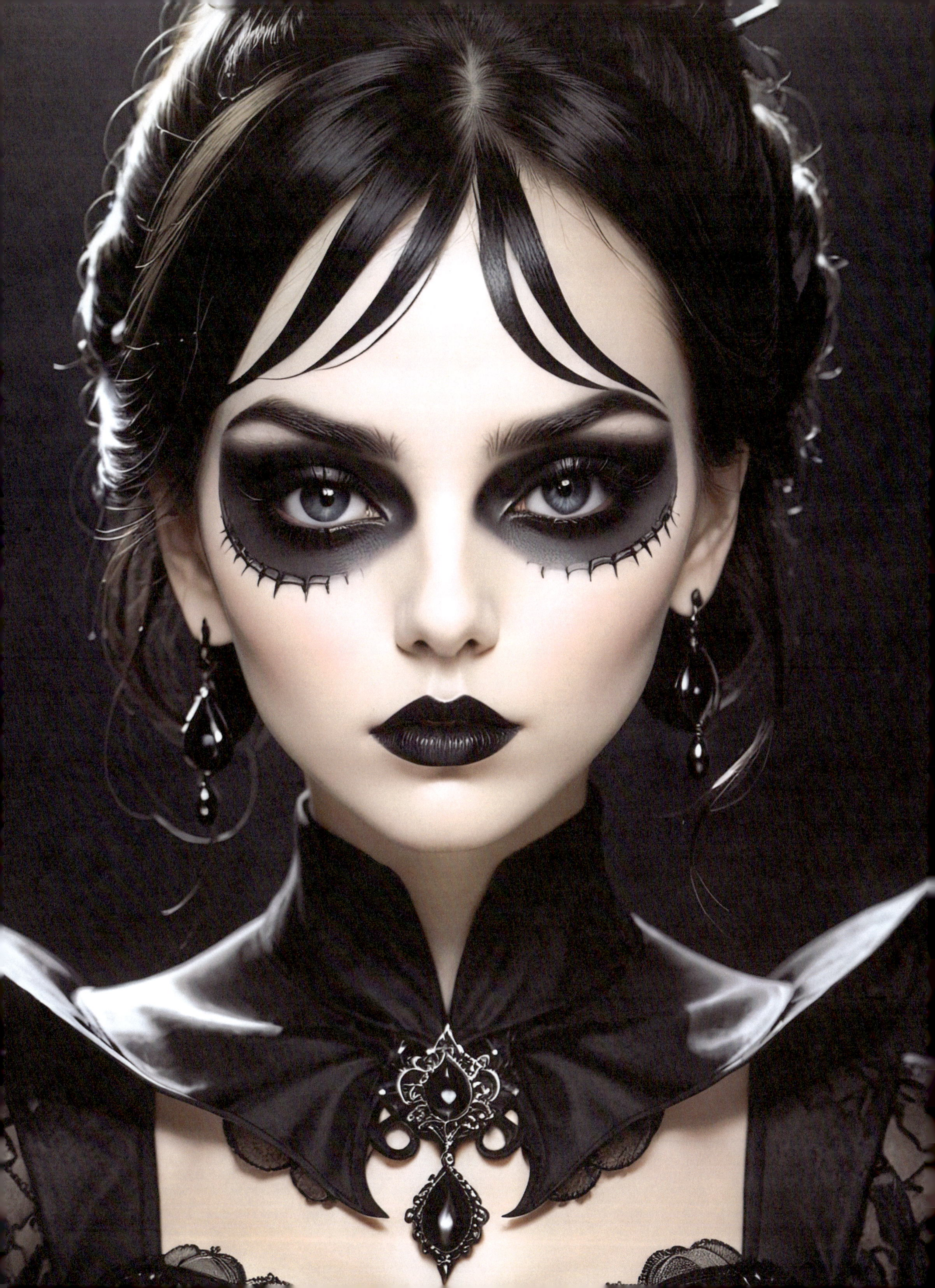

"ENCHANTRESS OF THE DARK WOODS"

STEP-BY-STEP INSTRUCTIONS:

1. SKIN PREPARATION:

TOOLS: LIGHT FOUNDATION, TRANSLUCENT POWDER.

INSTRUCTIONS: APPLY A LIGHT FOUNDATION ALL OVER THE FACE TO ACHIEVE A SMOOTH, EVEN COMPLEXION. ENSURE THE FOUNDATION IS EVENLY BLENDED, CREATING A PERFECT BASE FOR THE DARK AND MYSTERIOUS MAKEUP.

2. EYES:

TOOLS: BLACK EYESHADOW, DARK GREEN EYESHADOW, BLACK EYELINER, MASCARA, GREEN CONTACT LENSES.

INSTRUCTIONS: APPLY BLACK EYESHADOW ON THE EYELIDS, BLENDING IT TOWARDS THE OUTER CORNERS FOR A DEEP, SMOKY EFFECT. ADD DARK GREEN EYESHADOW TO THE CREASE AND LOWER LASH LINE TO INTRODUCE A HINT OF COLOR. USE BLACK EYELINER TO DRAW BOLD LINES ON THE UPPER LID AND EXTEND THEM SLIGHTLY FOR A DRAMATIC LOOK. APPLY MASCARA TO ENHANCE THE LASHES, THEN WEAR GREEN CONTACT LENSES TO GIVE THE EYES AN ENCHANTING, FOREST-LIKE GAZE.

3. EYEBROWS:

TOOLS: BLACK BROW PENCIL OR BLACK EYESHADOW.

INSTRUCTIONS: DEFINE THE EYEBROWS WITH A BLACK BROW PENCIL OR EYESHADOW, GIVING THEM A SHARP AND WELL-DEFINED SHAPE THAT COMPLEMENTS THE INTENSE EYE MAKEUP.

4. LIPS:

TOOLS: BLACK LIPSTICK.

INSTRUCTIONS: APPLY BLACK LIPSTICK CAREFULLY, OUTLINING THE LIPS FOR A BOLD AND STRIKING APPEARANCE. THE LIPS SHOULD LOOK DARK AND ALLURING, PERFECTLY MATCHING THE GOTHIC THEME.

5. FINISHING DETAILS:

TOOLS: BLACK LACE CHOKER, DARK GREEN GEMSTONE JEWELRY.

INSTRUCTIONS: ENHANCE THE LOOK WITH A BLACK LACE CHOKER AND JEWELRY ADORNED WITH DARK GREEN GEMSTONES TO MATCH THE EYE COLOR. THE ACCESSORIES SHOULD ADD AN ELEMENT OF ELEGANCE AND MYSTERY TO THE OVERALL APPEARANCE.

6. HAIR AND COSTUME:

TOOLS: BLACK WIG OR HAIR STYLED BLACK, GOTHIC DRESS, BLACK CAPE.

INSTRUCTIONS: COMPLETE THE LOOK BY WEARING A BLACK WIG OR STYLING THE HAIR IN LOOSE, DARK WAVES. ADD A GOTHIC DRESS AND A BLACK CAPE TO INTENSIFY THE AURA OF A MYSTERIOUS ENCHANTRESS LURKING IN THE DARK WOODS.

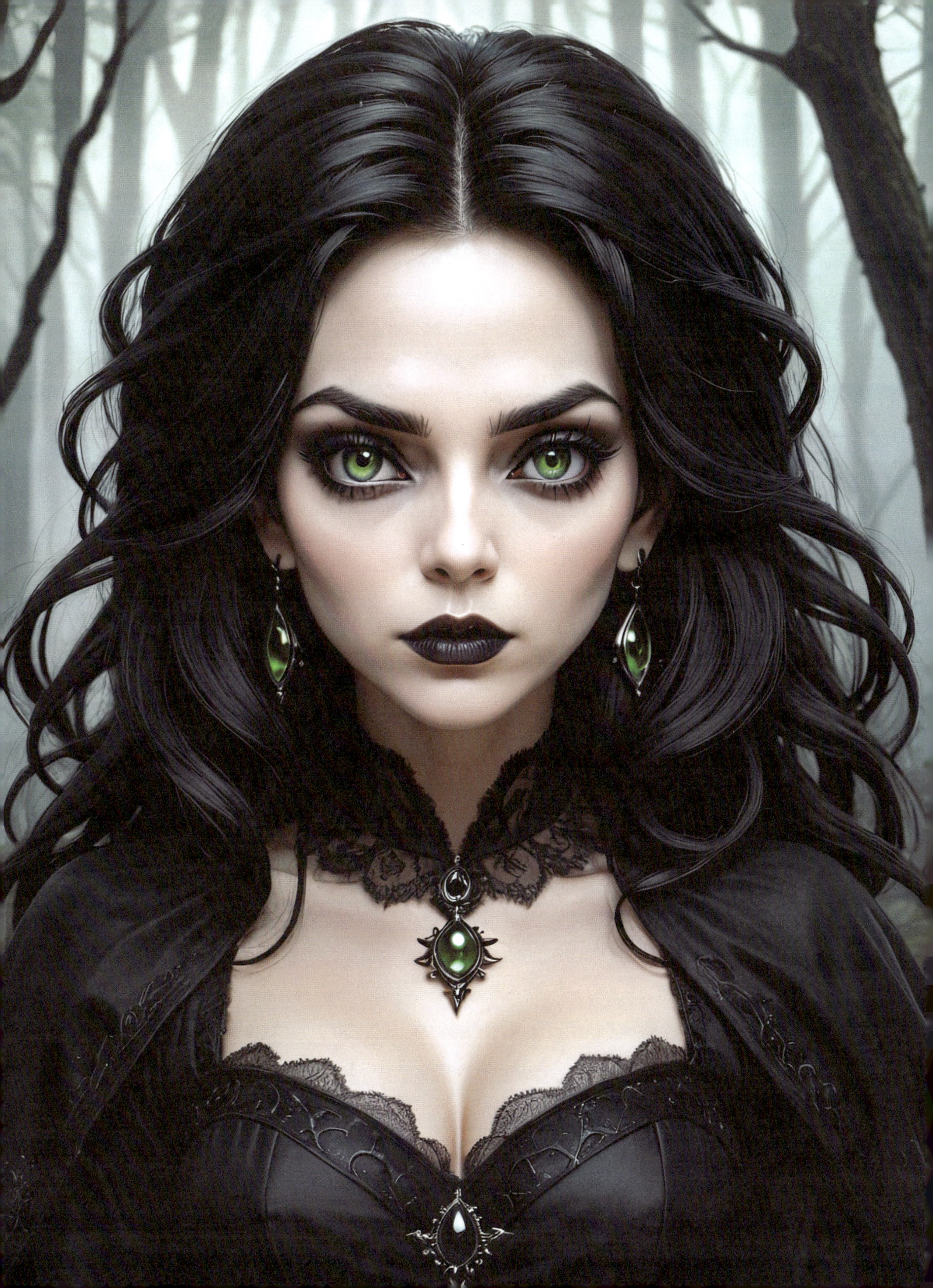

"GOTHIC VAMPIRE COUNTESS"

STEP-BY-STEP INSTRUCTIONS:

1. SKIN PREPARATION:

TOOLS: LIGHT FOUNDATION, TRANSLUCENT POWDER.

INSTRUCTIONS: APPLY A LIGHT FOUNDATION ALL OVER THE FACE TO CREATE A SMOOTH, PALE COMPLEXION. THIS WILL SERVE AS THE PERFECT BASE FOR THE GOTHIC VAMPIRE LOOK. SET THE FOUNDATION WITH TRANSLUCENT POWDER TO ENSURE A MATTE FINISH.

2. EYES:

TOOLS: DEEP RED AND BLACK EYESHADOW, BLACK EYELINER, MASCARA, AMBER OR RED CONTACT LENSES.

INSTRUCTIONS: START BY APPLYING DEEP RED EYESHADOW TO THE ENTIRE EYELID, BLENDING IT OUTWARDS TOWARDS THE TEMPLES. ADD BLACK EYESHADOW TO THE OUTER CORNERS AND CREASE TO CREATE DEPTH AND A SMOKY EFFECT. USE BLACK EYELINER TO DRAW A PRECISE LINE ON THE UPPER AND LOWER LASH LINES. APPLY MASCARA GENEROUSLY TO BOTH THE UPPER AND LOWER LASHES. FINISH THE EYE LOOK WITH AMBER OR RED CONTACT LENSES FOR AN INTENSE, HYPNOTIC GAZE.

3. EYEBROWS:

TOOLS: BLACK BROW PENCIL OR BLACK EYESHADOW.

INSTRUCTIONS: DEFINE THE EYEBROWS WITH A BLACK BROW PENCIL OR EYESHADOW, GIVING THEM A SHARP, DRAMATIC SHAPE THAT ENHANCES THE INTENSITY OF THE EYE MAKEUP.

4. LIPS:

TOOLS: DEEP RED OR BURGUNDY LIPSTICK.

INSTRUCTIONS: APPLY A DEEP RED OR BURGUNDY LIPSTICK, CAREFULLY OUTLINING THE LIPS FOR A BOLD AND SULTRY LOOK. THE LIPS SHOULD COMPLEMENT THE DRAMATIC EYES, ENHANCING THE OVERALL VAMPIRE AESTHETIC.

5. FINISHING DETAILS:

TOOLS: GOTHIC JEWELRY WITH RED GEMSTONES, BLACK LACE CHOKER.

INSTRUCTIONS: ACCESSORIZE WITH GOTHIC JEWELRY, SUCH AS EARRINGS AND A NECKLACE ADORNED WITH RED GEMSTONES. A BLACK LACE CHOKER WILL ADD ELEGANCE AND COMPLETE THE VAMPIRE COUNTESS LOOK.

6. HAIR AND COSTUME:

TOOLS: BLACK WIG OR HAIR STYLED BLACK WITH RED HIGHLIGHTS, GOTHIC DRESS, BLACK CAPE.

INSTRUCTIONS: STYLE THE HAIR IN LOOSE WAVES OR WEAR A BLACK WIG WITH SUBTLE RED HIGHLIGHTS TO ADD DIMENSION. CHOOSE A GOTHIC DRESS WITH INTRICATE LACE DETAILS AND A BLACK CAPE TO COMPLETE THE LOOK OF A SOPHISTICATED AND DEADLY VAMPIRE COUNTESS.

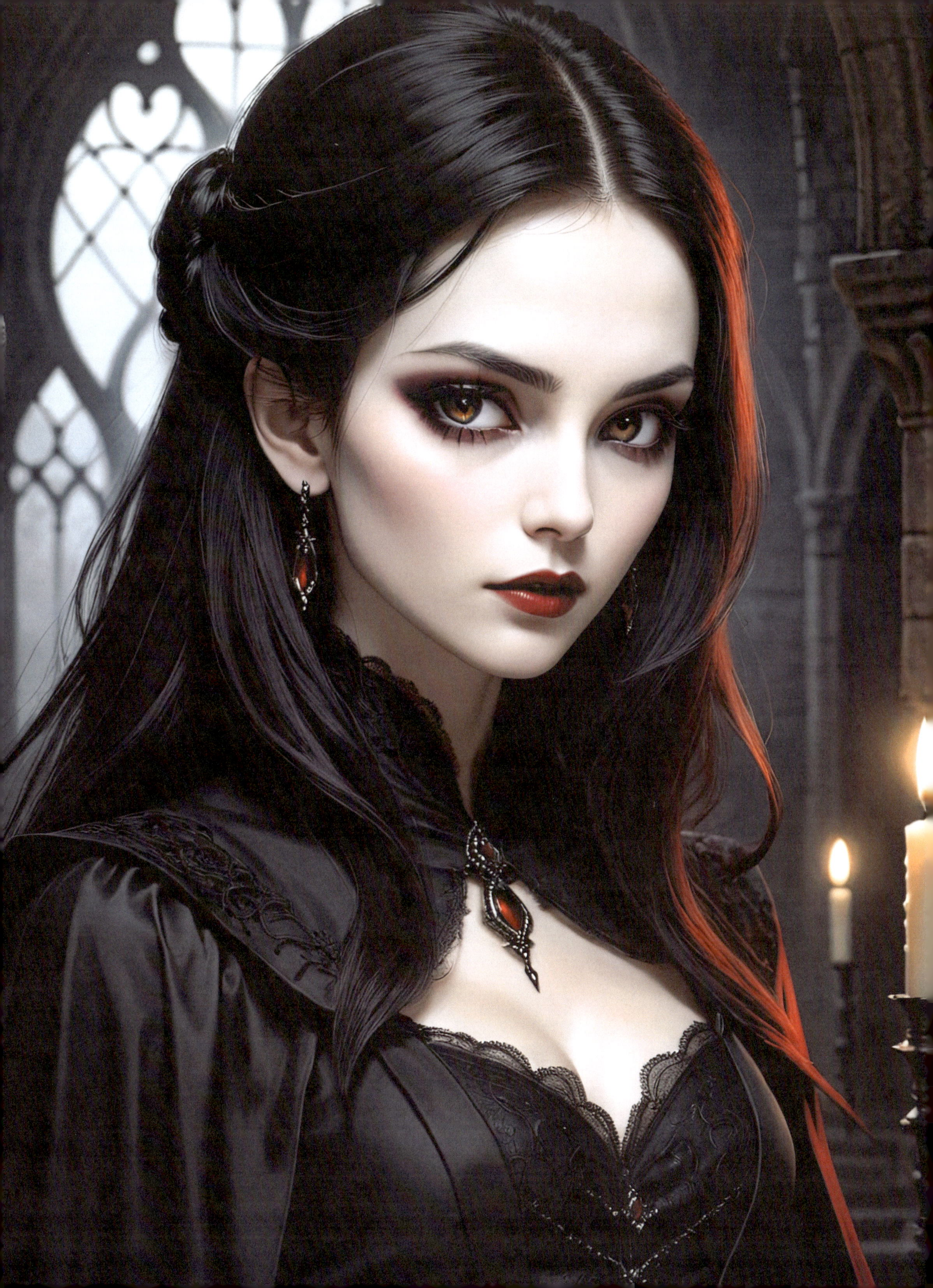

"THE CURSED UNDEAD"

STEP-BY-STEP INSTRUCTIONS:

1. SKIN PREPARATION:

TOOLS: PALE GREY FOUNDATION OR FACE PAINT, TRANSLUCENT POWDER.

INSTRUCTIONS: APPLY A PALE GREY FOUNDATION OR FACE PAINT TO THE ENTIRE FACE AND NECK TO CREATE A DEATHLY, UNDEAD COMPLEXION. ENSURE THE MAKEUP IS EVENLY BLENDED FOR A CONSISTENT, CORPSE-LIKE APPEARANCE. SET THE MAKEUP WITH TRANSLUCENT POWDER TO MAINTAIN THE MATTE FINISH.

2. EYES:

TOOLS: DARK PURPLE AND BLACK EYESHADOW, BLACK EYELINER, MASCARA, PURPLE CONTACT LENSES.

INSTRUCTIONS: APPLY DARK PURPLE EYESHADOW AROUND THE EYES, FOCUSING ON THE EYELIDS AND BLENDING IT DOWN TO THE LOWER LASH LINE TO CREATE A SUNKEN, HOLLOW LOOK. USE BLACK EYESHADOW TO DEEPEN THE EFFECT IN THE INNER CORNERS AND AROUND THE EYES. ADD BLACK EYELINER TO THE WATERLINE AND LASH LINES TO INTENSIFY THE HOLLOW GAZE. APPLY A FEW COATS OF MASCARA, FOCUSING ON THE UPPER AND LOWER LASHES. FINISH BY INSERTING PURPLE CONTACT LENSES TO GIVE THE EYES AN EERIE, SUPERNATURAL GLOW.

3. FACE DETAILING:

TOOLS: BLACK FACE PAINT, FINE BRUSH, PURPLE FACE PAINT (OPTIONAL).

INSTRUCTIONS: USE BLACK FACE PAINT TO DRAW FINE, VEIN-LIKE CRACKS EXTENDING FROM THE EYES, FOREHEAD, AND AROUND THE MOUTH, GIVING THE APPEARANCE OF DECAYED, CRACKING SKIN. OPTIONALLY, ADD SUBTLE TOUCHES OF PURPLE FACE PAINT WITHIN THE CRACKS FOR A MORE DETAILED AND EERIE EFFECT.

4. LIPS:

TOOLS: PALE PINK OR PURPLE LIPSTICK.

INSTRUCTIONS: APPLY A PALE PINK OR PURPLE LIPSTICK TO THE LIPS, KEEPING THE APPLICATION LIGHT TO GIVE A WITHERED AND LIFELESS APPEARANCE. SLIGHTLY SMUDGE THE EDGES FOR A MORE DISHEVELED, UNDEAD LOOK.

5. NECK AND CHEST DETAILING:

TOOLS: BLACK AND PURPLE FACE PAINT, FINE BRUSH.

INSTRUCTIONS: EXTEND THE VEIN-LIKE CRACKS DOWN THE NECK AND ONTO THE CHEST, CREATING THE ILLUSION OF A CURSE SPREADING THROUGH THE BODY. HIGHLIGHT CERTAIN AREAS WITH PURPLE PAINT TO EMPHASIZE THE EERIE, CURSED EFFECT.

6. HAIR AND COSTUME:

TOOLS: PURPLE WIG OR HAIR SPRAY, TATTERED CLOTHING.

INSTRUCTIONS: STYLE THE HAIR WITH A PURPLE WIG OR APPLY PURPLE HAIR SPRAY TO ADD A GHOSTLY, CURSED EFFECT. PAIR THE LOOK WITH TATTERED, WORN-OUT CLOTHING THAT COMPLEMENTS THE UNDEAD APPEARANCE. THE OVERALL LOOK SHOULD BE HAUNTING AND UNSETTLING, FITTING FOR A CURSED BEING RISEN FROM THE GRAVE.

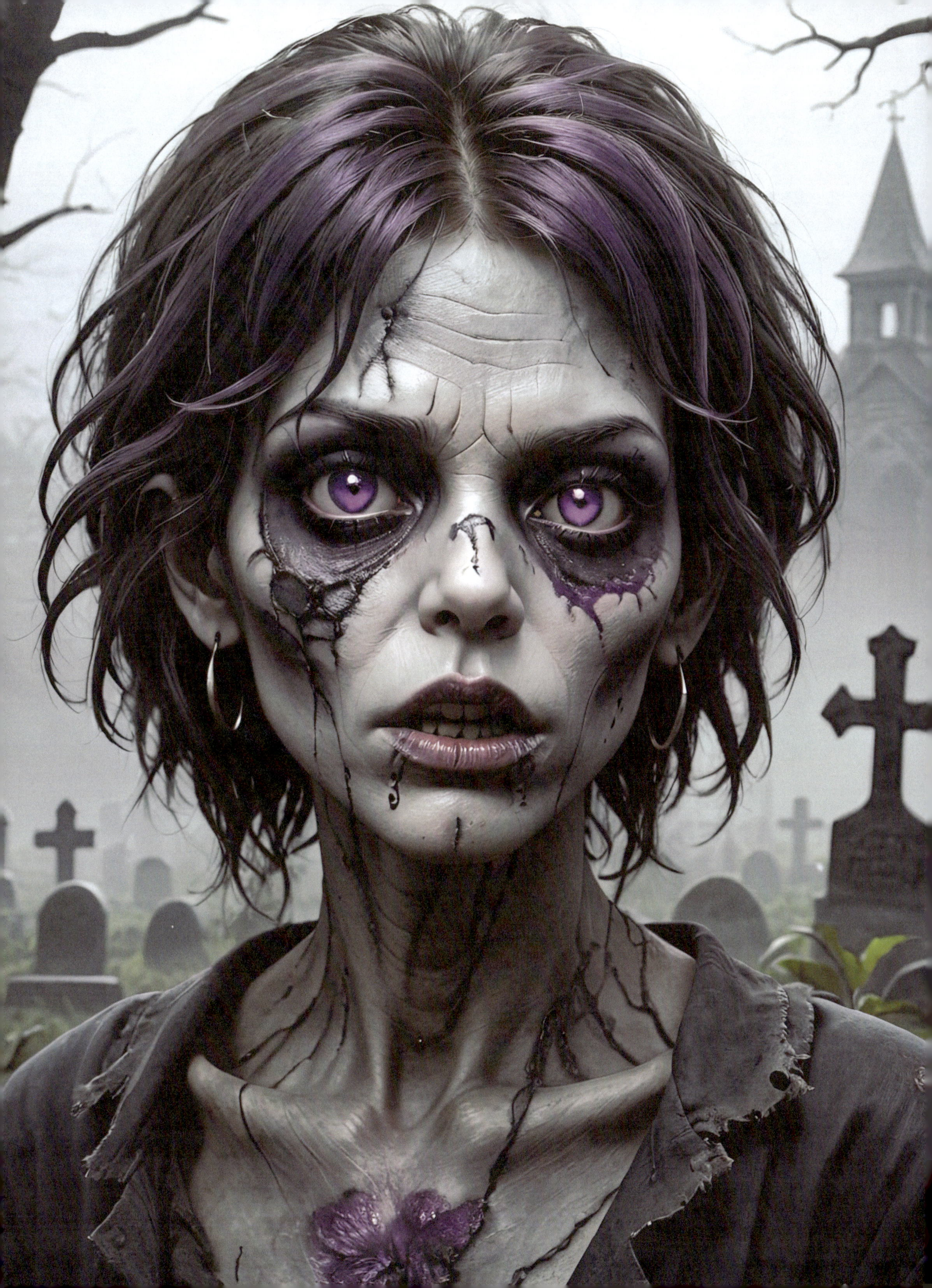

"THE DARK EMPRESS"

STEP-BY-STEP INSTRUCTIONS:

1. SKIN PREPARATION:

TOOLS: LIGHT FOUNDATION, TRANSLUCENT POWDER.

INSTRUCTIONS: APPLY A LIGHT FOUNDATION ACROSS THE FACE TO CREATE A FLAWLESS, PORCELAIN-LIKE COMPLEXION. SET THE FOUNDATION WITH TRANSLUCENT POWDER TO ACHIEVE A SMOOTH AND MATTE FINISH.

2. EYES:

TOOLS: BLACK AND DEEP RED EYESHADOW, BLACK EYELINER, MASCARA, LIGHT BLUE CONTACT LENSES.

INSTRUCTIONS: START BY APPLYING BLACK EYESHADOW AROUND THE EYES, FOCUSING ON THE EYELIDS AND BLENDING IT OUTWARDS TO CREATE A DRAMATIC WINGED EFFECT. ADD DEEP RED EYESHADOW TO THE CREASE AND BLEND IT INTO THE BLACK FOR ADDED DEPTH. USE BLACK EYELINER TO DRAW PRECISE LINES ALONG THE UPPER AND LOWER LASH LINES, EXTENDING SLIGHTLY FOR AN INTENSE, CAT-EYE EFFECT. APPLY MASCARA GENEROUSLY TO ENHANCE THE LASHES. FINISH BY INSERTING LIGHT BLUE CONTACT LENSES TO GIVE THE EYES A PIERCING, OTHERWORLDLY GAZE.

3. FACE DETAILING:

TOOLS: BLACK FACE PAINT, FINE BRUSH.

INSTRUCTIONS: USE BLACK FACE PAINT TO CREATE INTRICATE, SYMMETRICAL DESIGNS ON THE FOREHEAD AND AROUND THE EYES. THESE DESIGNS SHOULD BE ELEGANT AND GOTHIC, RESEMBLING ORNATE FILIGREE OR FLAMES. THE PATTERNS SHOULD EXTEND SLIGHTLY ONTO THE CHEEKS, FRAMING THE EYES AND ENHANCING THE OVERALL DARK, REGAL APPEARANCE.

4. LIPS:

TOOLS: DEEP RED LIPSTICK.

INSTRUCTIONS: APPLY A DEEP RED LIPSTICK TO THE LIPS, CAREFULLY DEFINING THE EDGES FOR A BOLD, SOPHISTICATED LOOK. THE LIPS SHOULD BE STRIKING AND COMPLEMENT THE DARK EYE MAKEUP.

5. HAIR AND FLORAL ACCENTS:

TOOLS: BLACK HAIR OR WIG, PURPLE FLOWERS.

INSTRUCTIONS: STYLE THE HAIR IN AN ELEGANT UPDO OR USE A BLACK WIG TO ACHIEVE A SLEEK LOOK. ADORN THE HAIR WITH PURPLE FLOWERS, PLACING THEM STRATEGICALLY TO ADD A TOUCH OF CONTRAST AND ELEGANCE TO THE DARK EMPRESS AESTHETIC.

6. COSTUME AND ACCESSORIES:

TOOLS: BLACK AND GOLD ARMOR-STYLE COSTUME, RED GEMSTONE JEWELRY.

INSTRUCTIONS: WEAR A BLACK AND GOLD ARMOR-STYLE COSTUME THAT EXUDES POWER AND AUTHORITY. ADD RED GEMSTONE JEWELRY, SUCH AS A STATEMENT NECKLACE AND MATCHING EARRINGS, TO COMPLETE THE LOOK. THE OVERALL OUTFIT SHOULD BE LUXURIOUS AND REGAL, FITTING FOR AN EMPRESS OF DARKNESS.

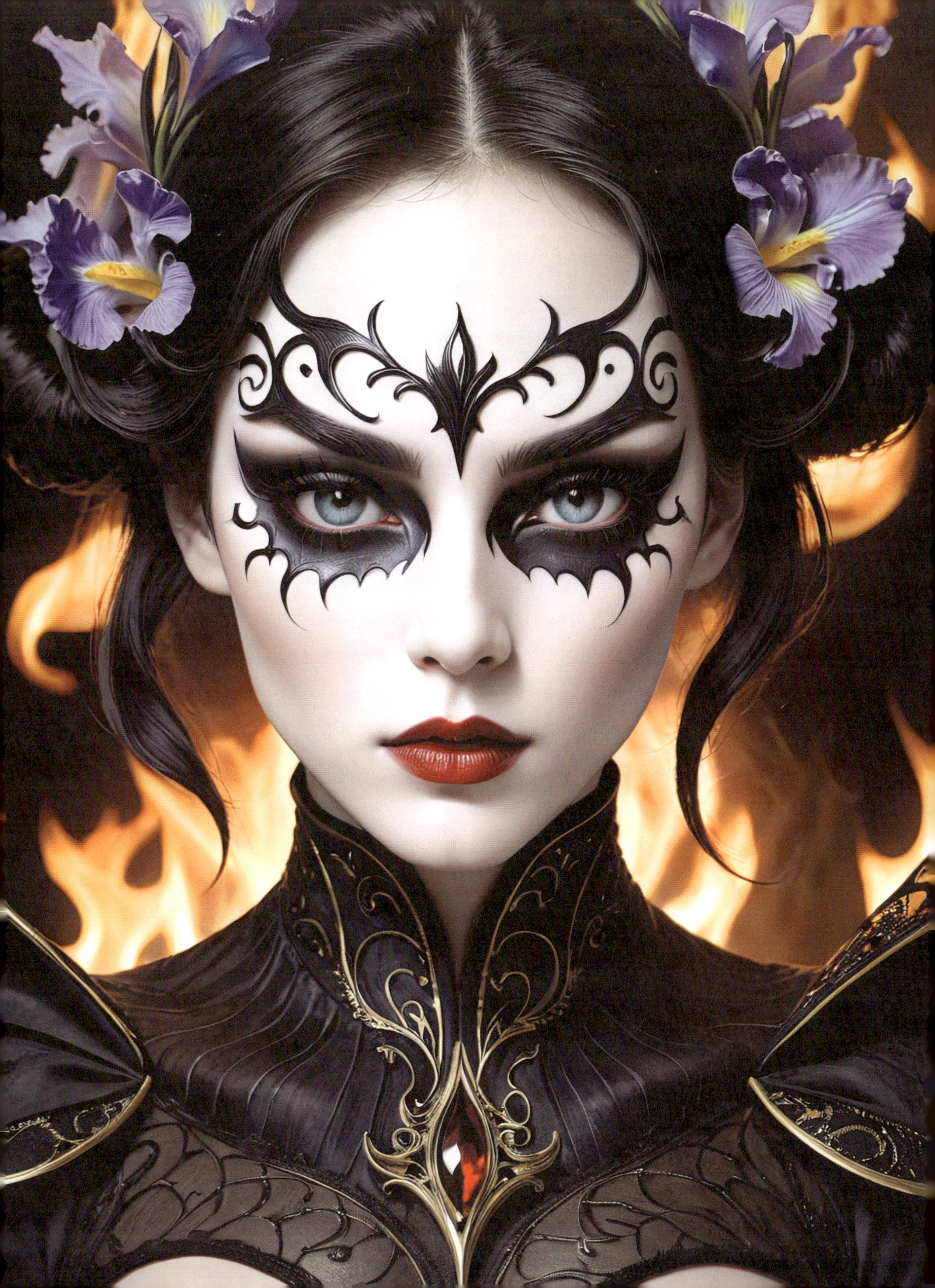

"ENCHANTED FOREST FELINE"

STEP-BY-STEP INSTRUCTIONS:

1. SKIN PREPARATION:

TOOLS: LIGHT FOUNDATION, TRANSLUCENT POWDER.

INSTRUCTIONS: BEGIN BY APPLYING A LIGHT FOUNDATION TO THE ENTIRE FACE TO CREATE A SMOOTH, EVEN BASE. SET THE FOUNDATION WITH TRANSLUCENT POWDER TO ENSURE A FLAWLESS FINISH.

2. EYES:

TOOLS: BLACK AND WHITE FACE PAINT, BLACK EYELINER, MASCARA, GREEN CONTACT LENSES.

INSTRUCTIONS: USE BLACK FACE PAINT TO CREATE A BOLD, FELINE-INSPIRED DESIGN AROUND THE EYES. EXTEND THE BLACK PAINT IN A WINGED SHAPE FROM THE INNER CORNERS TO THE TEMPLES. ADD WHITE FACE PAINT ABOVE THE BROWS AND BELOW THE EYES, FORMING STYLIZED STRIPES THAT RESEMBLE A CAT'S MARKINGS. USE BLACK EYELINER TO LINE THE EYES, CREATING A DRAMATIC, CAT-EYE EFFECT. APPLY MASCARA TO THE LASHES FOR ADDED VOLUME AND DEFINITION. INSERT GREEN CONTACT LENSES TO GIVE THE EYES A MYSTICAL, FELINE APPEARANCE.

3. FACE DETAILING:

TOOLS: BLACK FACE PAINT, FINE BRUSH, WHITE FACE PAINT.

INSTRUCTIONS: USE BLACK FACE PAINT TO DRAW A SMALL, FELINE-LIKE NOSE AT THE TIP OF THE NOSE. ADD DELICATE WHITE DOTS AROUND THE LOWER EYES TO MIMIC WHISKER SPOTS. ENSURE THE DETAILS ARE SYMMETRICAL AND WELL-DEFINED.

4. LIPS:

TOOLS: BLACK LIPSTICK.

INSTRUCTIONS: APPLY BLACK LIPSTICK TO THE LIPS, DEFINING THE SHAPE SHARPLY TO MATCH THE OVERALL FELINE THEME. THE LIPS SHOULD APPEAR SLEEK AND POLISHED, COMPLEMENTING THE DRAMATIC EYE MAKEUP.

5. HAIR AND ACCESSORIES:

TOOLS: BLACK WIG OR HAIR STYLED WITH CAT EARS, YELLOW FEATHER EARRINGS.

INSTRUCTIONS: STYLE THE HAIR WITH A BLACK WIG OR ADD CAT EAR ACCESSORIES FOR AN AUTHENTIC FELINE LOOK. COMPLETE THE LOOK WITH YELLOW FEATHER EARRINGS THAT ADD A POP OF COLOR AND ENHANCE THE MYSTICAL FOREST CREATURE VIBE.

6. COSTUME:

TOOLS: BLACK OR ANIMAL PRINT COSTUME.

INSTRUCTIONS: PAIR THE MAKEUP WITH A BLACK OR ANIMAL PRINT COSTUME THAT EMPHASIZES THE FELINE FEATURES. THE OVERALL LOOK SHOULD BE BOTH ELEGANT AND WILD, CAPTURING THE ESSENCE OF AN ENCHANTED FOREST FELINE.

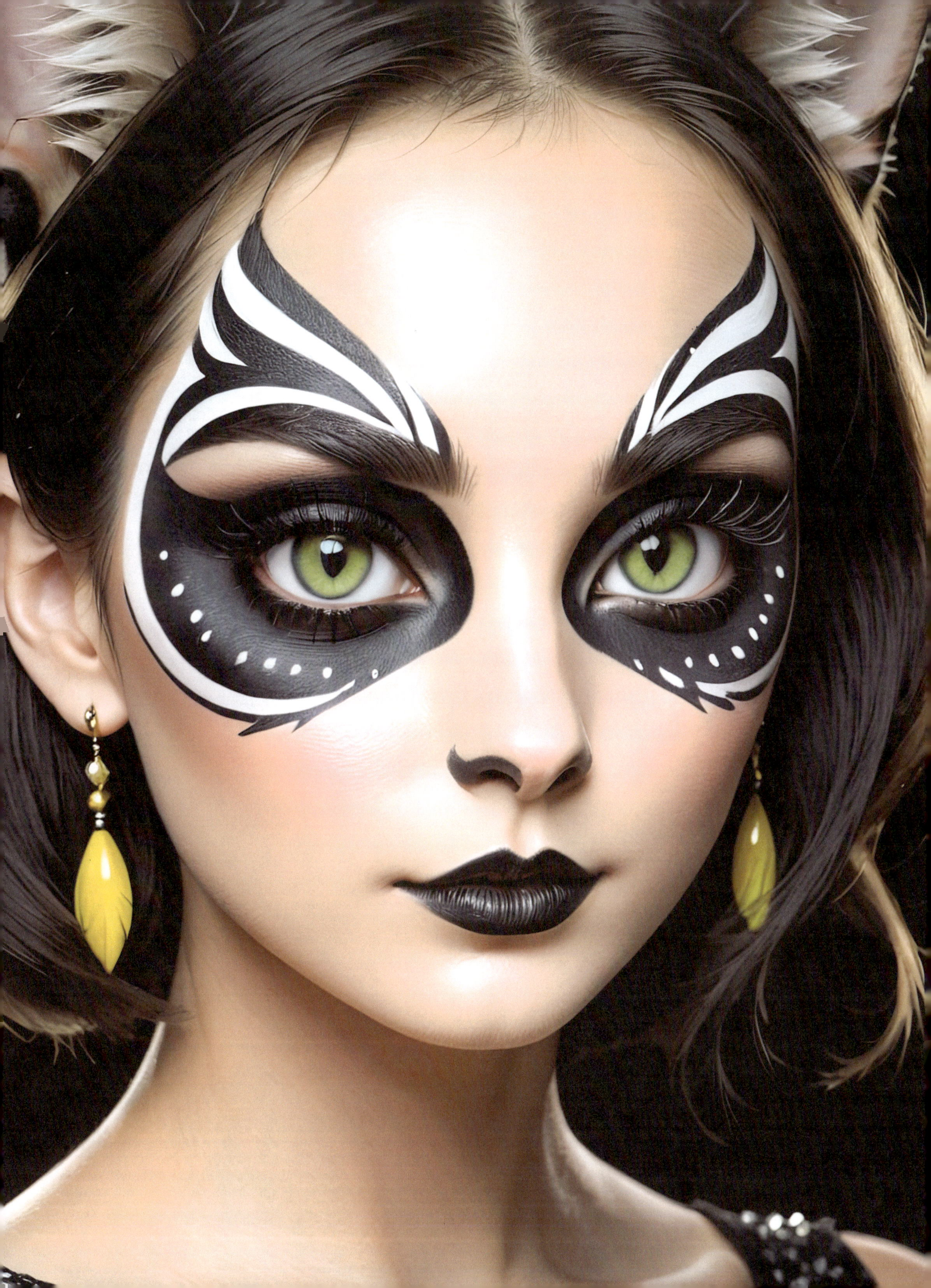

"TWISTED JESTER"

STEP-BY-STEP INSTRUCTIONS:

1. SKIN PREPARATION:

TOOLS: WHITE FACE PAINT, TRANSLUCENT POWDER.

INSTRUCTIONS: APPLY WHITE FACE PAINT EVENLY ACROSS THE ENTIRE FACE TO CREATE A SMOOTH, OPAQUE BASE. THIS WILL GIVE THE FACE A PALE, THEATRICAL APPEARANCE ESSENTIAL FOR THE JESTER LOOK. SET THE FACE PAINT WITH TRANSLUCENT POWDER TO PREVENT SMUDGING AND ENSURE LONG-LASTING WEAR.

2. EYES:

TOOLS: BLACK AND PURPLE EYESHADOW, BLACK FACE PAINT, BLACK EYELINER, MASCARA, GREY CONTACT LENSES.

INSTRUCTIONS: BEGIN BY APPLYING PURPLE EYESHADOW TO THE EYELIDS, BLENDING IT UPWARDS TOWARDS THE BROW BONE FOR A SMOKY EFFECT. USE BLACK EYESHADOW TO DARKEN THE CREASE AND OUTER CORNERS OF THE EYES. NEXT, USE BLACK FACE PAINT TO CREATE INTRICATE, SYMMETRICAL DESIGNS AROUND THE EYES, RESEMBLING JESTER MAKEUP. LINE THE EYES WITH BLACK EYELINER, ENSURING THE LINES ARE SHARP AND DEFINED. APPLY MASCARA TO THE LASHES TO ENHANCE THE EYES FURTHER. FINISH WITH GREY CONTACT LENSES TO GIVE THE EYES AN EERIE, MISCHIEVOUS LOOK.

3. FACE DETAILING:

TOOLS: BLACK FACE PAINT, FINE BRUSH.

INSTRUCTIONS: USING BLACK FACE PAINT AND A FINE BRUSH, CREATE DETAILED, CURVED LINES EXTENDING FROM THE EYE DESIGNS TOWARDS THE CHEEKS AND FOREHEAD. THE DESIGNS SHOULD BE SHARP AND SYMMETRICAL, ENHANCING THE JESTER THEME. ADD A SMALL BLACK DIAMOND SHAPE TO THE CENTER OF THE FOREHEAD TO COMPLETE THE LOOK.

4. LIPS:

TOOLS: BLACK LIPSTICK.

INSTRUCTIONS: APPLY BLACK LIPSTICK TO THE LIPS, CAREFULLY OUTLINING AND FILLING THEM IN FOR A BOLD, DRAMATIC LOOK. THE LIPS SHOULD BE STRIKING AND MATCH THE DARK TONES OF THE EYE MAKEUP.

5. HAIR AND ACCESSORIES:

TOOLS: JESTER HAT WITH HORNS, BLACK AND GOLD EARRINGS.

INSTRUCTIONS: WEAR A JESTER HAT WITH CURVED HORNS, PREFERABLY IN PURPLE TO MATCH THE EYE MAKEUP. THE HAT SHOULD BE PROMINENT AND ADD A WHIMSICAL YET TWISTED ELEMENT TO THE LOOK. ADD BLACK AND GOLD EARRINGS TO COMPLEMENT THE OUTFIT AND ENHANCE THE OVERALL APPEARANCE.

6. COSTUME:

TOOLS: JESTER COSTUME IN BLACK, WHITE, AND GOLD.

INSTRUCTIONS: PAIR THE MAKEUP WITH A TRADITIONAL JESTER COSTUME, INCORPORATING BLACK, WHITE, AND GOLD COLORS. THE COSTUME SHOULD BE THEATRICAL, WITH RUFFLES, STRIPES, AND BOLD PATTERNS THAT ECHO THE INTRICATE MAKEUP DESIGN.

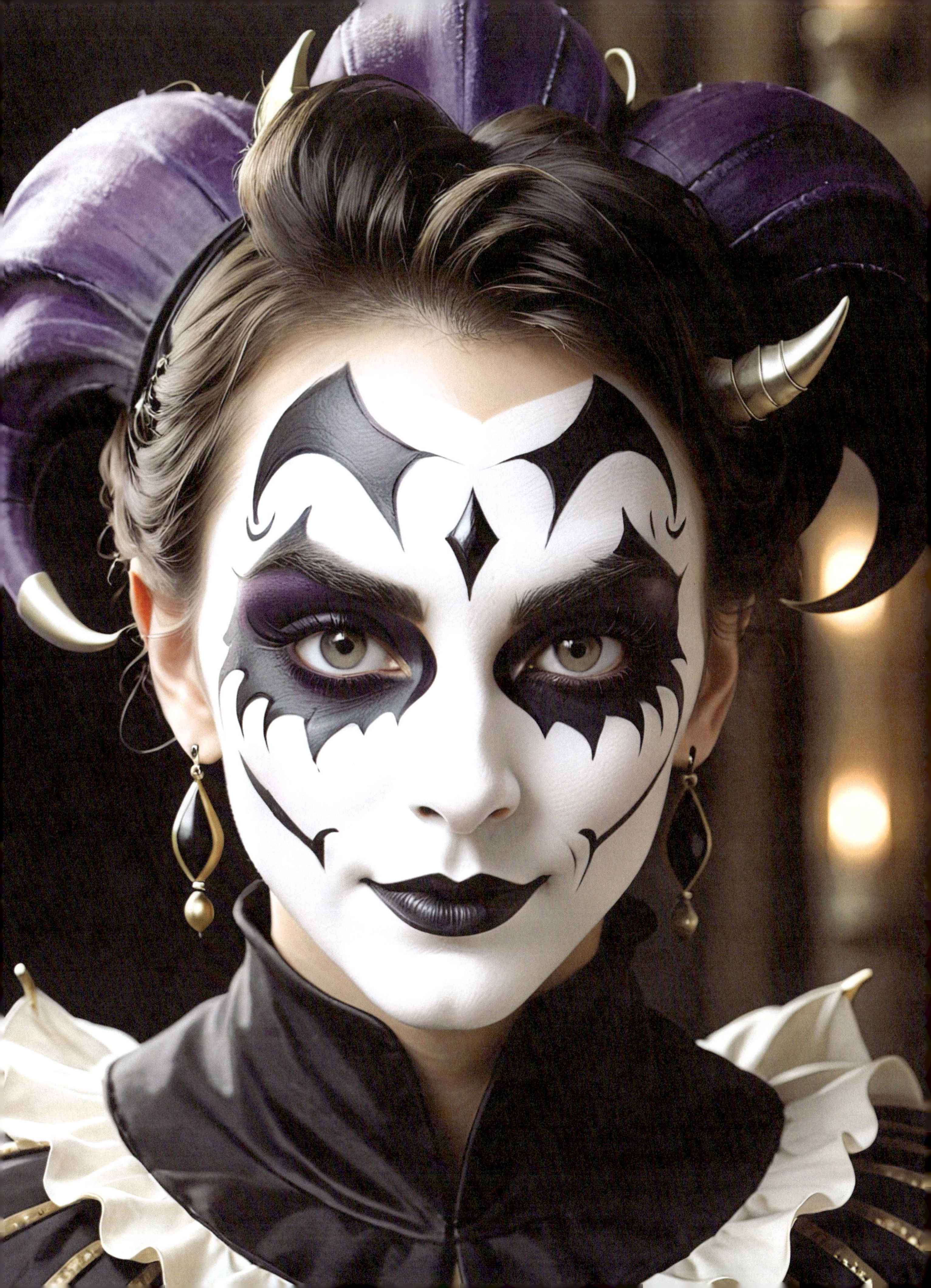

"SHADOW ENCHANTRESS"

STEP-BY-STEP INSTRUCTIONS:

1. SKIN PREPARATION:

TOOLS: LIGHT FOUNDATION, TRANSLUCENT POWDER.

INSTRUCTIONS: APPLY A LIGHT FOUNDATION TO CREATE A SMOOTH AND EVEN COMPLEXION. SET THE FOUNDATION WITH TRANSLUCENT POWDER TO MAINTAIN A MATTE FINISH THAT ALLOWS THE OTHER MAKEUP ELEMENTS TO STAND OUT.

2. EYES:

TOOLS: DARK GREY AND BLACK EYESHADOW, BLACK EYELINER, MASCARA, LIGHT BLUE CONTACT LENSES.

INSTRUCTIONS: START BY APPLYING DARK GREY EYESHADOW ACROSS THE EYELIDS AND BLENDING IT OUTWARDS TO CREATE A SMOKY EFFECT. ADD BLACK EYESHADOW TO THE CREASE AND OUTER CORNERS TO DEEPEN THE LOOK. USE BLACK EYELINER TO DEFINE THE LASH LINES, EXTENDING SLIGHTLY BEYOND THE OUTER CORNERS FOR A DRAMATIC EFFECT. APPLY MASCARA TO ENHANCE THE LASHES, MAKING THEM BOLD AND VOLUMINOUS. FINISH BY INSERTING LIGHT BLUE CONTACT LENSES TO GIVE THE EYES A COLD, ETHEREAL GAZE.

3. FACE DETAILING:

TOOLS: BLACK AND GREY FACE PAINT, FINE BRUSH.

INSTRUCTIONS: USE BLACK AND GREY FACE PAINT TO CREATE ELEGANT, CURVED DESIGNS AROUND THE EYES AND ON THE FOREHEAD. THE PATTERNS SHOULD RESEMBLE SWIRLING SHADOWS, ADDING AN AIR OF MYSTERY AND ENCHANTMENT TO THE FACE. ENSURE THE DESIGNS ARE SYMMETRICAL AND SMOOTHLY BLENDED FOR A SEAMLESS APPEARANCE.

4. LIPS:

TOOLS: NUDE OR PALE PINK LIPSTICK.

INSTRUCTIONS: APPLY A NUDE OR PALE PINK LIPSTICK TO KEEP THE LIPS SUBTLE AND UNDERSTATED. THIS HELPS TO DRAW ATTENTION TO THE EYES AND THE INTRICATE FACE DESIGNS.

5. HAIR AND ACCESSORIES:

TOOLS: LOOSE BLACK HAIR OR WIG, BLACK FEATHER EARRINGS.

INSTRUCTIONS: STYLE THE HAIR LOOSELY WITH SOFT WAVES OR USE A BLACK WIG FOR AN EFFORTLESSLY ELEGANT LOOK. PAIR WITH BLACK FEATHER EARRINGS TO ENHANCE THE ETHEREAL, DARK ENCHANTRESS VIBE.

6. COSTUME:

TOOLS: BLACK FEATHERED OR GOTHIC-INSPIRED DRESS.

INSTRUCTIONS: COMPLETE THE LOOK WITH A BLACK FEATHERED OR GOTHIC-INSPIRED DRESS. THE OUTFIT SHOULD BE DARK AND FLOWING, ADDING TO THE MYSTERIOUS AND ENCHANTING AURA OF THE SHADOW ENCHANTRESS.

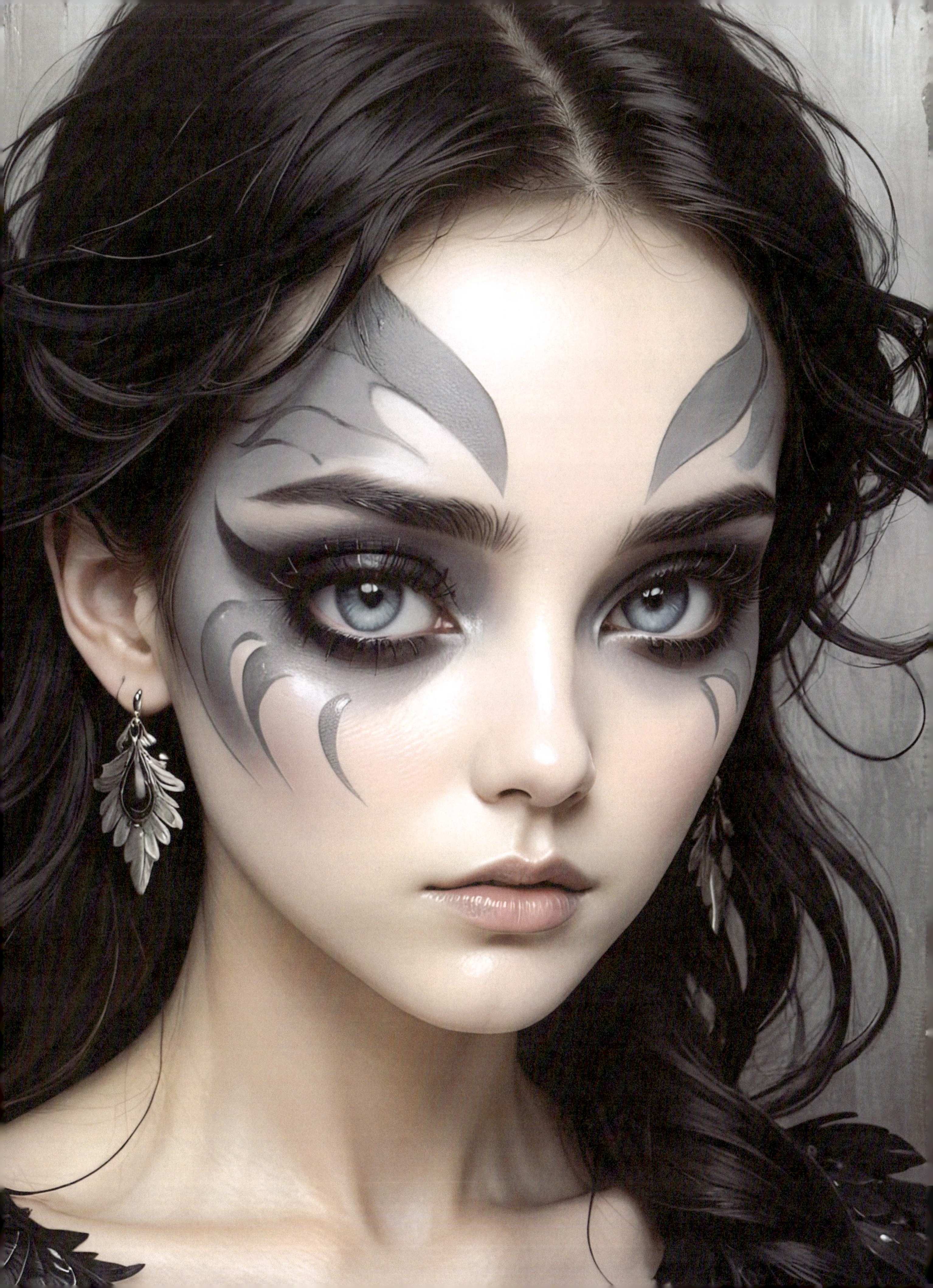

"MYSTICAL NIGHT WOLF"

STEP-BY-STEP INSTRUCTIONS:

1. SKIN PREPARATION:

TOOLS: LIGHT FOUNDATION, TRANSLUCENT POWDER.

INSTRUCTIONS: APPLY A LIGHT FOUNDATION TO CREATE A SMOOTH AND FLAWLESS BASE. SET THE FOUNDATION WITH TRANSLUCENT POWDER TO ENSURE THE MAKEUP STAYS IN PLACE AND MAINTAINS A MATTE FINISH.

2. EYES:

TOOLS: BLACK AND BLUE FACE PAINT, BLACK EYELINER, MASCARA, YELLOW CONTACT LENSES.

INSTRUCTIONS: USE BLACK FACE PAINT TO CREATE A MASK-LIKE DESIGN AROUND THE EYES, EXTENDING IT TOWARDS THE TEMPLES AND SLIGHTLY DOWN THE CHEEKS. ADD BLUE FACE PAINT ALONG THE EDGES OF THE MASK, INCORPORATING INTRICATE TRIBAL-LIKE PATTERNS TO GIVE THE DESIGN A MYSTICAL FEEL. LINE THE EYES WITH BLACK EYELINER, ENSURING THE LINES ARE SHARP AND DEFINED. APPLY MASCARA TO ENHANCE THE LASHES AND ADD DRAMA TO THE EYES. FINISH WITH YELLOW CONTACT LENSES TO GIVE THE EYES A PIERCING, WOLF-LIKE APPEARANCE.

3. FACE DETAILING:

TOOLS: BLACK AND BLUE FACE PAINT, FINE BRUSH.

INSTRUCTIONS: USE A FINE BRUSH AND BLUE FACE PAINT TO ADD ADDITIONAL DETAILING WITHIN THE MASK, FOCUSING ON THE CENTER OF THE FOREHEAD AND AROUND THE EYES. THE DESIGNS SHOULD RESEMBLE ANCIENT RUNES OR TRIBAL MARKINGS, ENHANCING THE MYSTICAL AND POWERFUL AURA OF THE WOLF. ENSURE THE DETAILING IS SYMMETRICAL AND PRECISE.

4. LIPS:

TOOLS: DARK GREY LIPSTICK.

INSTRUCTIONS: APPLY DARK GREY LIPSTICK TO THE LIPS, KEEPING THE COLOR INTENSE YET MUTED TO COMPLEMENT THE BOLD EYE MAKEUP. THE LIPS SHOULD APPEAR SLEEK AND POLISHED.

5. HAIR AND ACCESSORIES:

TOOLS: WOLF EARS, BLACK AND BLUE FEATHER EARRINGS, MATCHING CHOKER.

INSTRUCTIONS: WEAR A PAIR OF REALISTIC WOLF EARS TO ADD AUTHENTICITY TO THE LOOK. PAIR THE EARS WITH BLACK AND BLUE FEATHER EARRINGS AND A MATCHING CHOKER TO ENHANCE THE MYSTICAL, NATURE-INSPIRED THEME OF THE MAKEUP.

6. COSTUME:

TOOLS: BLACK OR GREY FUR-LINED COSTUME.

INSTRUCTIONS: COMPLETE THE LOOK WITH A FUR-LINED COSTUME IN BLACK OR GREY TONES. THE OUTFIT SHOULD BE REMINISCENT OF A POWERFUL WOLF, EMPHASIZING STRENGTH AND CONNECTION TO NATURE.

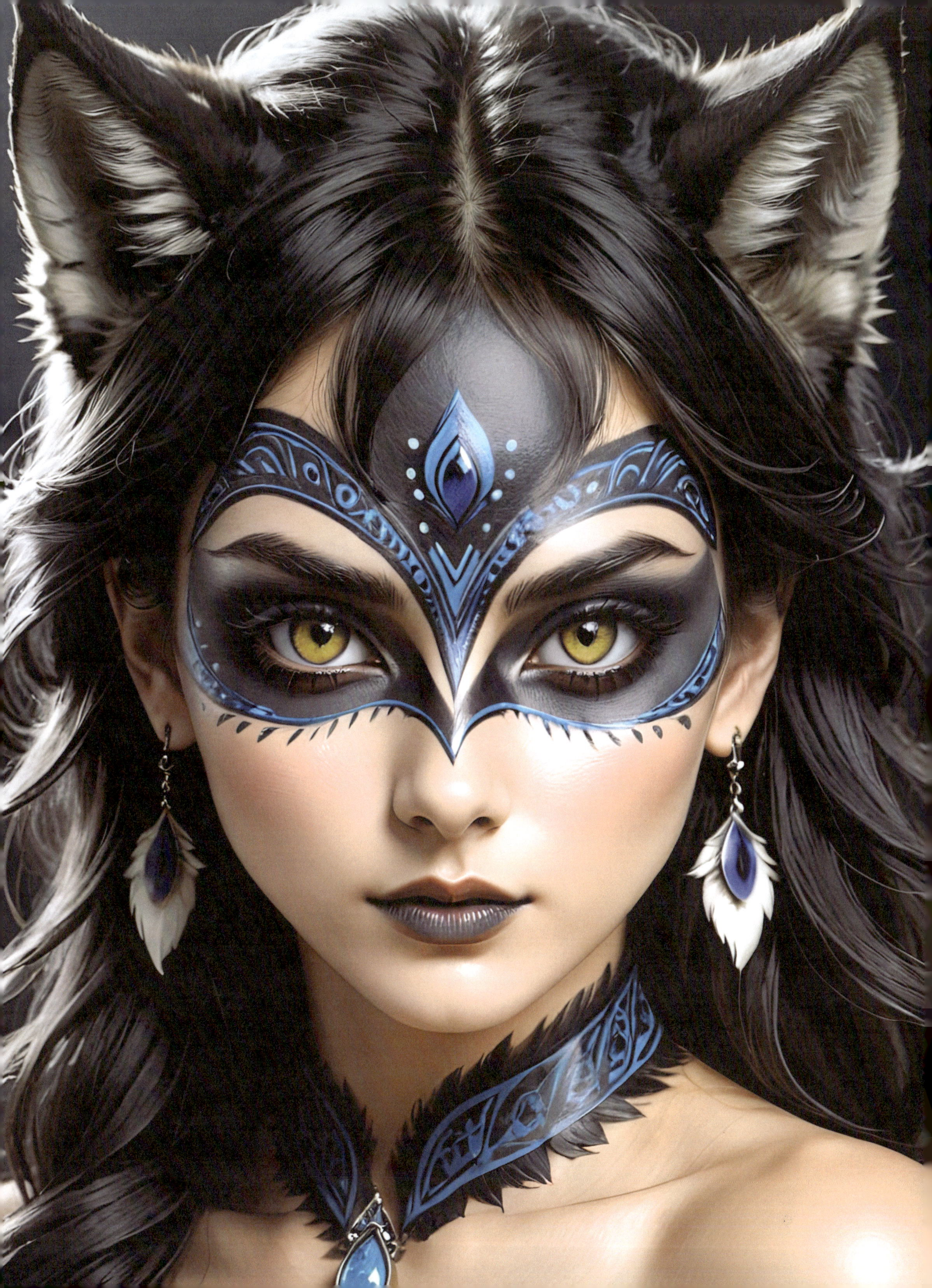

"ETHEREAL GHOST QUEEN"

STEP-BY-STEP INSTRUCTIONS:

1. SKIN PREPARATION:

TOOLS: WHITE FOUNDATION, TRANSLUCENT POWDER.

INSTRUCTIONS: START BY APPLYING A WHITE FOUNDATION EVENLY ACROSS THE FACE AND NECK TO CREATE A GHOSTLY PALE BASE. SET THE FOUNDATION WITH TRANSLUCENT POWDER TO ENSURE THE MAKEUP REMAINS SMOOTH AND MATTE THROUGHOUT.

2. EYES:

TOOLS: BLACK AND GREY EYESHADOW, BLACK EYELINER, MASCARA, LIGHT GREY CONTACT LENSES.

INSTRUCTIONS: APPLY GREY EYESHADOW OVER THE EYELIDS, BLENDING IT TOWARDS THE OUTER CORNERS AND INTO THE CREASE. USE BLACK EYESHADOW AROUND THE EDGES TO ADD DEPTH AND CREATE A HOLLOW, HAUNTING LOOK. LINE THE EYES WITH BLACK EYELINER, EXTENDING SLIGHTLY BEYOND THE OUTER CORNERS FOR A DRAMATIC EFFECT. APPLY MASCARA TO ENHANCE THE LASHES. FINISH BY INSERTING LIGHT GREY CONTACT LENSES TO GIVE THE EYES A COLD, ETHEREAL GAZE.

3. FACE DETAILING:

TOOLS: BLACK AND GREY FACE PAINT, FINE BRUSH.

INSTRUCTIONS: USE BLACK AND GREY FACE PAINT TO CREATE DELICATE PATTERNS ON THE FOREHEAD AND CHEEKS. THE DESIGNS SHOULD RESEMBLE THE ELEGANT, DECAYED BEAUTY OF AN ANCIENT QUEEN, WITH SYMMETRICAL SHAPES AND FADED DETAILS THAT EVOKE A SENSE OF TIMELESSNESS. FOCUS ON BLENDING THE EDGES TO CREATE A SOFT, GHOSTLY APPEARANCE.

4. LIPS:

TOOLS: DARK GREY LIPSTICK.

INSTRUCTIONS: APPLY DARK GREY LIPSTICK TO THE LIPS, KEEPING THE COLOR MUTED TO COMPLEMENT THE OVERALL GHOSTLY THEME. THE LIPS SHOULD APPEAR SUBTLE YET DEFINED.

5. HAIR AND ACCESSORIES:

TOOLS: WHITE OR SILVER WIG, ANTIQUE-STYLE EARRINGS.

INSTRUCTIONS: STYLE THE HAIR IN LOOSE WAVES OR USE A WHITE OR SILVER WIG TO ADD AN ETHEREAL TOUCH. PAIR WITH ANTIQUE-STYLE EARRINGS TO ENHANCE THE REGAL AND OTHERWORLDLY APPEARANCE OF THE GHOST QUEEN.

6. COSTUME:

TOOLS: GREY OR SILVER LACE GOWN, LACE CHOKER.

INSTRUCTIONS: COMPLETE THE LOOK WITH A FLOWING GREY OR SILVER LACE GOWN THAT ADDS TO THE GHOSTLY, ELEGANT THEME. PAIR WITH A LACE CHOKER TO EMPHASIZE THE ROYAL ASPECT OF THE CHARACTER.

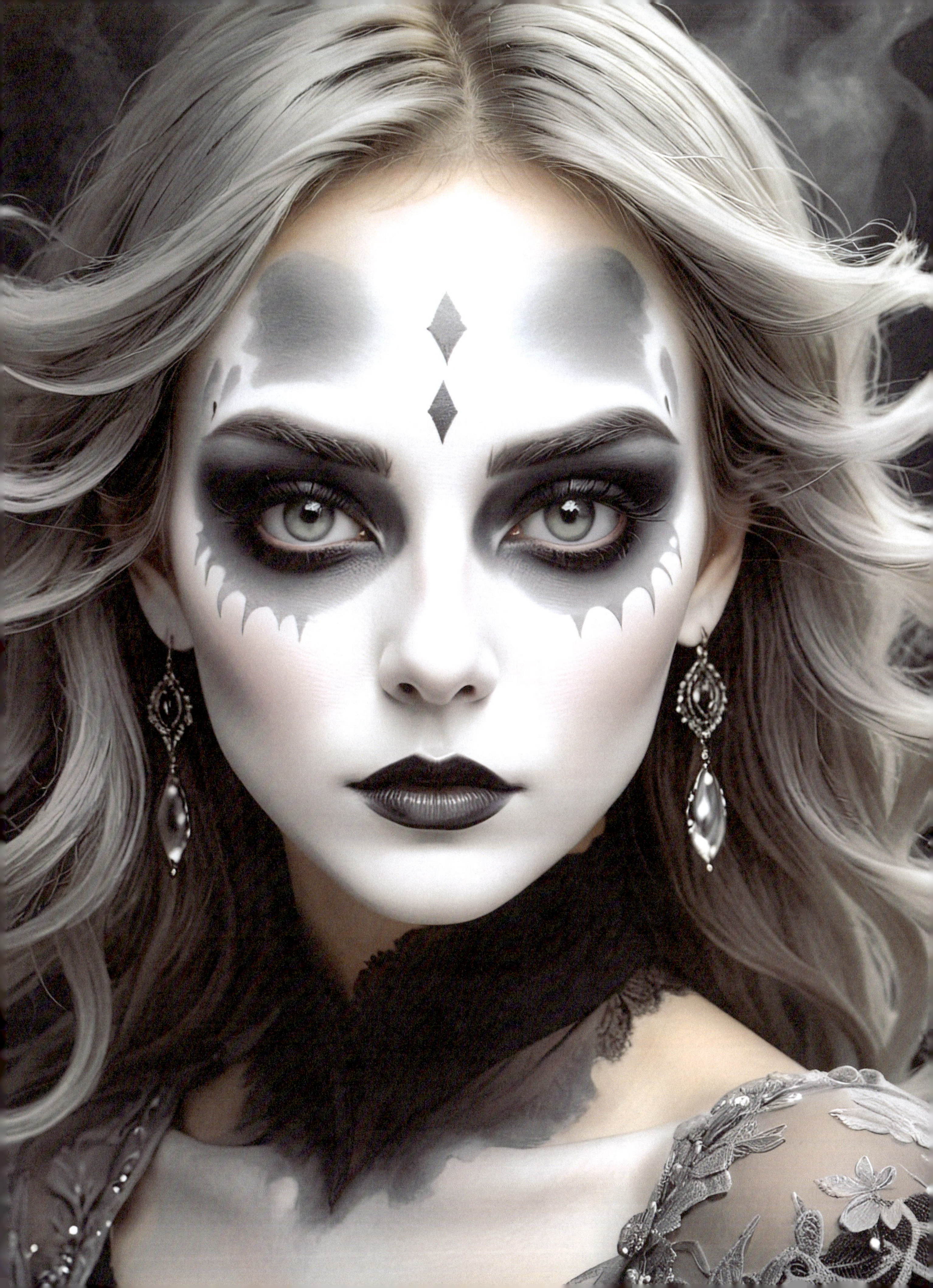

"GOTHIC FAIRY PRINCESS"

STEP-BY-STEP INSTRUCTIONS:

1. SKIN PREPARATION:

TOOLS: WHITE FOUNDATION, TRANSLUCENT POWDER.

INSTRUCTIONS: BEGIN BY APPLYING A WHITE FOUNDATION TO CREATE A PORCELAIN-LIKE COMPLEXION. ENSURE THE APPLICATION IS EVEN ACROSS THE FACE, NECK, AND SHOULDERS. SET THE FOUNDATION WITH TRANSLUCENT POWDER TO MAINTAIN A MATTE FINISH.

2. EYES:

TOOLS: BLACK AND GREY EYESHADOW, BLACK EYELINER, MASCARA, LIGHT GREY CONTACT LENSES.

INSTRUCTIONS: APPLY GREY EYESHADOW OVER THE ENTIRE EYELID, EXTENDING IT SLIGHTLY BEYOND THE OUTER CORNERS TO CREATE A SOFT, SMOKY EFFECT. USE BLACK EYESHADOW TO DEEPEN THE CREASE AND ALONG THE LOWER LASH LINE. LINE THE EYES WITH BLACK EYELINER, BOTH ON THE UPPER AND LOWER WATERLINES, TO ENHANCE THE DRAMATIC LOOK. APPLY A GENEROUS COAT OF MASCARA TO THE LASHES. FINISH WITH LIGHT GREY CONTACT LENSES TO GIVE THE EYES AN OTHERWORLDLY, FAIRY-LIKE APPEARANCE.

3. FACE DETAILING:

TOOLS: WHITE AND BLACK FACE PAINT, FINE BRUSH.

INSTRUCTIONS: USING A FINE BRUSH AND WHITE FACE PAINT, CREATE DELICATE, INTRICATE DESIGNS ON THE FOREHEAD AND AROUND THE EYES, REMINISCENT OF LACE OR FLORAL PATTERNS. ADD SMALL BLACK DETAILS TO CONTRAST AND ENHANCE THE WHITE DESIGNS, ENSURING THE OVERALL LOOK IS SYMMETRICAL AND ELEGANT.

4. LIPS:

TOOLS: DARK PLUM LIPSTICK.

INSTRUCTIONS: APPLY DARK PLUM LIPSTICK TO THE LIPS, KEEPING THE EDGES SHARP AND DEFINED. THE COLOR SHOULD BE RICH YET MUTED TO MATCH THE ETHEREAL THEME OF THE LOOK.

5. HAIR AND ACCESSORIES:

TOOLS: HAIRPINS, ARTIFICIAL FLOWERS, BLACK CHOKER, EARRINGS.

INSTRUCTIONS: STYLE THE HAIR IN A NEAT UPDO, SECURING IT WITH HAIRPINS. ADD ARTIFICIAL FLOWERS TO THE HAIR, FOCUSING ON SOFT COLORS LIKE WHITE OR LIGHT GREY TO COMPLEMENT THE MAKEUP. PAIR WITH A BLACK LACE CHOKER AND DELICATE EARRINGS TO COMPLETE THE GOTHIC FAIRY AESTHETIC.

6. COSTUME:

TOOLS: LACE OR SILK GOWN, TRANSPARENT WINGS.

INSTRUCTIONS: CHOOSE A GOWN MADE OF LACE OR SILK IN SOFT GREY OR WHITE TONES TO KEEP THE LOOK COHESIVE. ADD A PAIR OF TRANSPARENT FAIRY WINGS TO COMPLETE THE TRANSFORMATION INTO A GOTHIC FAIRY PRINCESS.

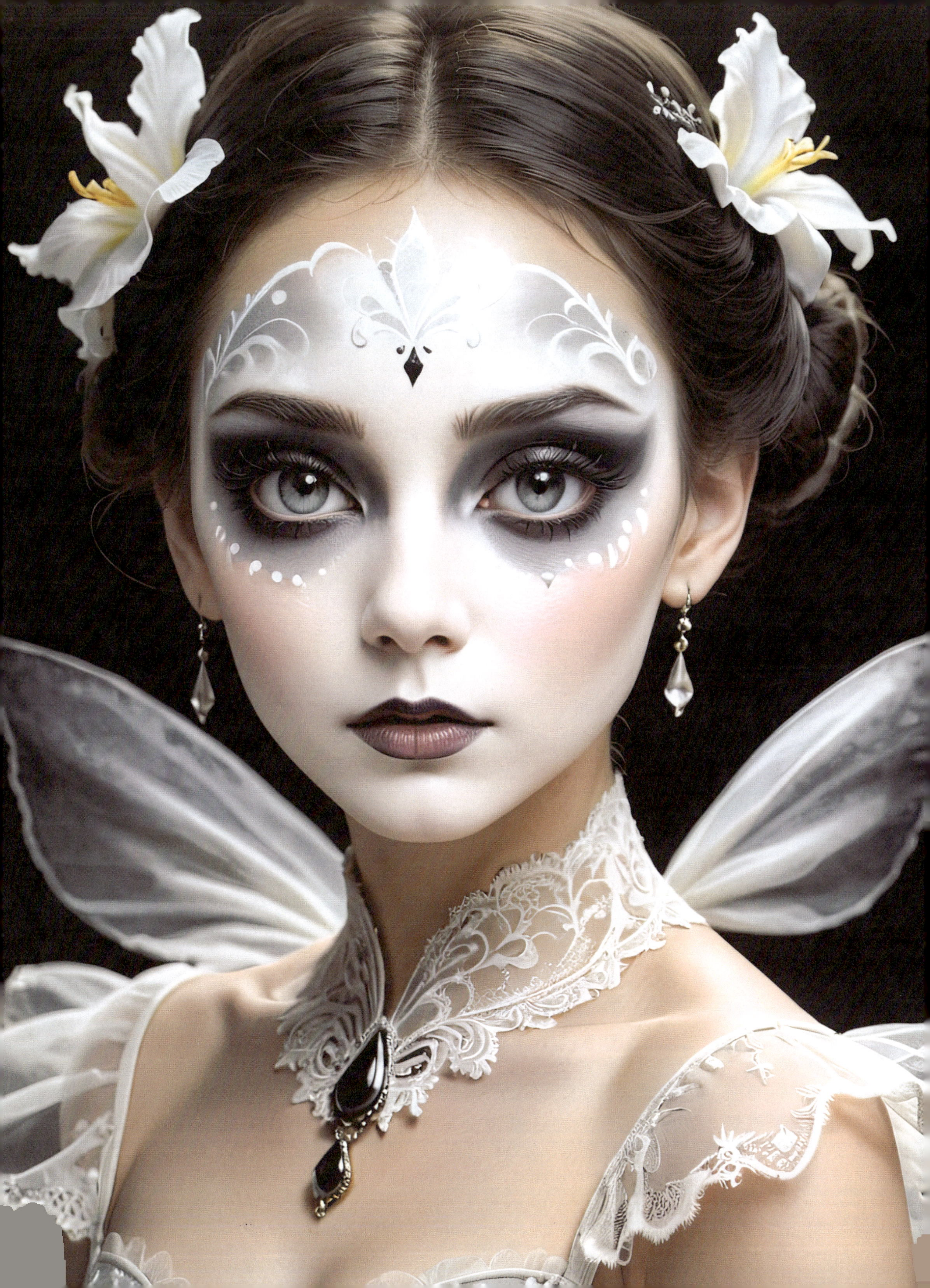

"INFERNO DEMONESS"

STEP-BY-STEP INSTRUCTIONS:

1. SKIN PREPARATION:

TOOLS: WHITE FOUNDATION, SETTING POWDER.

INSTRUCTIONS: START BY APPLYING A WHITE FOUNDATION OVER THE ENTIRE FACE, NECK, AND ANY VISIBLE SKIN AREAS TO CREATE A GHOSTLY BASE. SET THE FOUNDATION WITH SETTING POWDER TO ENSURE IT STAYS MATTE AND LONG-LASTING.

2. EYES:

TOOLS: BLACK AND ORANGE EYESHADOW, BLACK EYELINER, MASCARA, AMBER CONTACT LENSES.

INSTRUCTIONS: APPLY BLACK EYESHADOW TO THE EYELIDS, EXTENDING IT OUTWARDS TO CREATE A WINGED EFFECT. ADD ORANGE EYESHADOW TO THE INNER CORNERS OF THE EYES, BLENDING IT INTO THE BLACK FOR A FIERY GRADIENT. LINE THE EYES WITH BLACK EYELINER, CREATING A BOLD WINGED LINE. APPLY MASCARA TO BOTH THE UPPER AND LOWER LASHES. FINISH WITH AMBER CONTACT LENSES TO GIVE THE EYES A BURNING, OTHERWORLDLY APPEARANCE.

3. FACE DETAILING:

TOOLS: BLACK AND ORANGE FACE PAINT, FINE BRUSHES.

INSTRUCTIONS: USING BLACK FACE PAINT AND A FINE BRUSH, CREATE FLAME-LIKE DESIGNS THAT START AT THE OUTER CORNERS OF THE EYES AND EXTEND ACROSS THE FOREHEAD AND CHEEKS. INCORPORATE ORANGE PAINT TO ENHANCE THE FLAME EFFECT, BLENDING IT INTO THE BLACK FOR A SMOLDERING LOOK. MAKE SURE THE DESIGNS ARE SYMMETRICAL AND MIRROR THE INTENSITY OF REAL FLAMES.

4. LIPS:

TOOLS: ORANGE LIPSTICK.

INSTRUCTIONS: APPLY A BOLD ORANGE LIPSTICK TO THE LIPS, KEEPING THE EDGES SHARP AND DEFINED TO MATCH THE FIERY THEME.

5. HAIR AND ACCESSORIES:

TOOLS: BLACK HAIR DYE OR WIG, ORANGE EXTENSIONS, BLACK HORNS, FLAME-LIKE EARRINGS.

INSTRUCTIONS: STYLE THE HAIR IN AN UPDO OR USE A BLACK WIG, ADDING ORANGE EXTENSIONS TO MIMIC THE LOOK OF FLAMES. ATTACH BLACK HORNS TO THE HEAD, POSITIONING THEM SECURELY. FINISH THE LOOK WITH FLAME-LIKE EARRINGS THAT ADD TO THE OVERALL INTENSITY.

6. COSTUME:

TOOLS: BLACK AND ORANGE ARMOR OR DRESS.

INSTRUCTIONS: CHOOSE A BLACK AND ORANGE COSTUME, PREFERABLY WITH SHARP, ANGULAR DETAILS THAT RESEMBLE FLAMES OR DEMONIC ARMOR. THE COSTUME SHOULD COMPLEMENT THE FIERY MAKEUP AND CONTRIBUTE TO THE OVERALL APPEARANCE OF THE INFERNO DEMONESS.

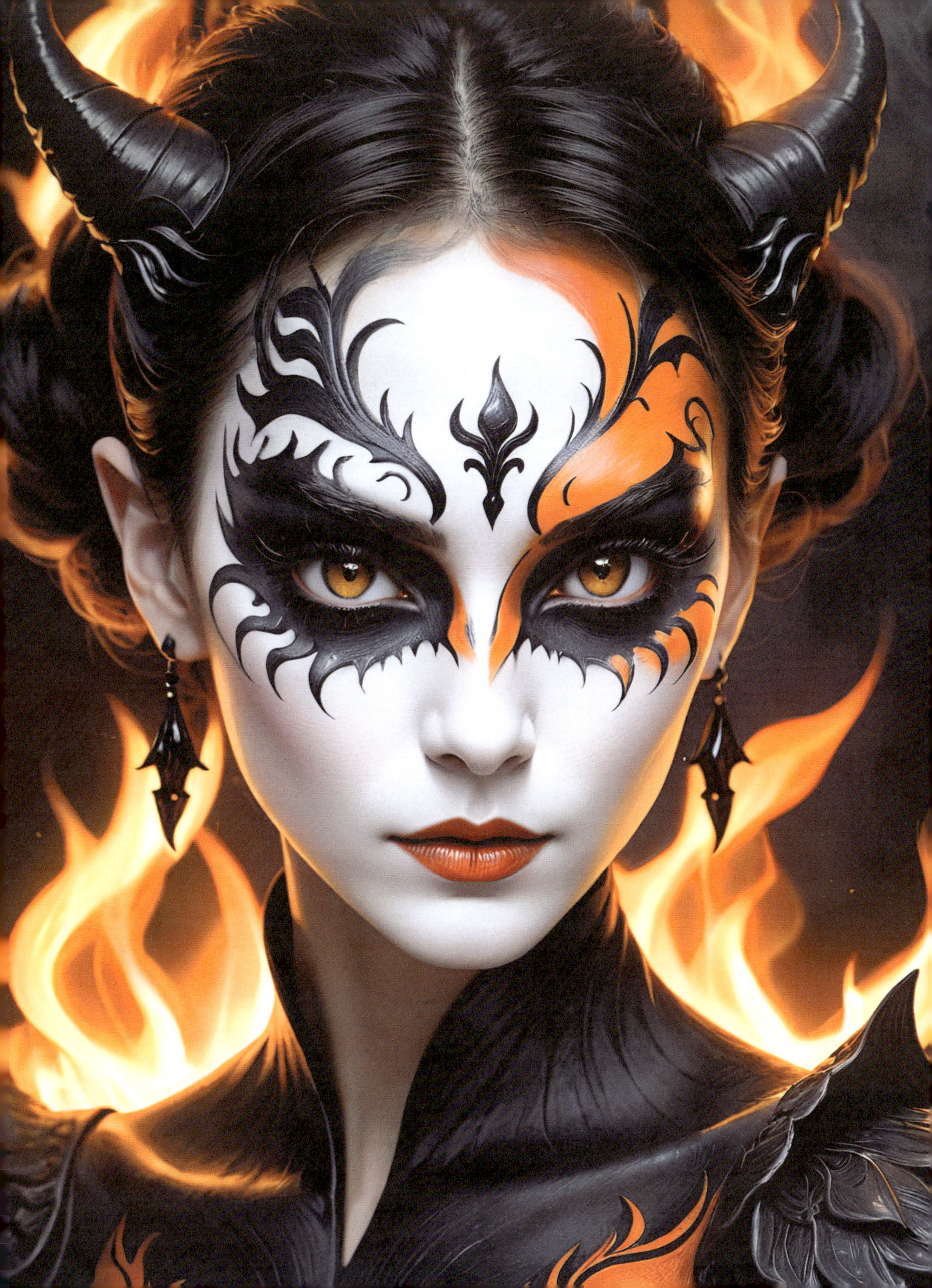

"SPIDER QUEEN"

STEP-BY-STEP INSTRUCTIONS:

1. SKIN PREPARATION:

TOOLS: PALE FOUNDATION, SETTING POWDER.

INSTRUCTIONS: BEGIN BY APPLYING A PALE FOUNDATION TO THE FACE AND NECK, CREATING A SMOOTH AND EVEN BASE. SET THE FOUNDATION WITH SETTING POWDER TO ENSURE A MATTE FINISH THAT WILL HOLD THE MAKEUP IN PLACE.

2. EYES:

TOOLS: BLUE AND BLACK EYESHADOW, BLACK EYELINER, MASCARA, LIGHT BLUE CONTACT LENSES.

INSTRUCTIONS: APPLY BLUE EYESHADOW TO THE EYELIDS, BLENDING UPWARDS TOWARDS THE BROW BONE. ADD BLACK EYESHADOW TO THE OUTER CORNERS OF THE EYES TO CREATE DEPTH AND A SMOKY EFFECT. USE BLACK EYELINER TO DEFINE THE EYES, EXTENDING THE LINE INTO A SHARP WING. APPLY MASCARA TO BOTH UPPER AND LOWER LASHES. LIGHT BLUE CONTACT LENSES WILL GIVE THE EYES AN ICY, SPIDER-LIKE APPEARANCE.

3. FACE DETAILING:

TOOLS: BLACK FACE PAINT, FINE BRUSHES, SILVER HIGHLIGHTER.

INSTRUCTIONS: USE BLACK FACE PAINT AND A FINE BRUSH TO DRAW A SPIDER WEB DESIGN STARTING FROM THE FOREHEAD AND EXTENDING OUTWARDS OVER THE FOREHEAD AND TEMPLES. ENSURE THE LINES ARE THIN AND PRECISE TO MIMIC THE DELICATE STRUCTURE OF A REAL SPIDER WEB. HIGHLIGHT THE WEB WITH SILVER HIGHLIGHTER TO GIVE IT A METALLIC, ETHEREAL SHEEN.

4. LIPS:

TOOLS: DEEP RED LIPSTICK.

INSTRUCTIONS: APPLY A DEEP RED LIPSTICK TO THE LIPS, KEEPING THE EDGES CRISP AND DEFINED. THE BOLD LIP COLOR CONTRASTS BEAUTIFULLY WITH THE COOL TONES OF THE EYE MAKEUP AND THE WEB DESIGN.

5. HAIR AND ACCESSORIES:

TOOLS: RED HAIR DYE OR WIG, SPIDER-SHAPED HAIRPINS, CRYSTAL EARRINGS.

INSTRUCTIONS: STYLE THE HAIR IN SOFT WAVES, EITHER USING A RED WIG OR DYEING THE HAIR A DEEP RED. PIN THE HAIR BACK SLIGHTLY WITH SPIDER-SHAPED HAIRPINS, ALLOWING SOME STRANDS TO FRAME THE FACE. FINISH WITH CRYSTAL EARRINGS THAT REFLECT THE BLUE TONES IN THE MAKEUP.

6. COSTUME:

TOOLS: BLACK SPIDER-THEMED BODYSUIT, SPIDER BROOCH.

INSTRUCTIONS: DRESS IN A BLACK BODYSUIT THAT FEATURES A SPIDER OR WEB DESIGN. ADD A SPIDER BROOCH AT THE COLLAR OR ON THE CHEST TO ENHANCE THE THEME. THE COSTUME SHOULD COMPLEMENT THE INTRICATE MAKEUP AND GIVE THE APPEARANCE OF A REGAL SPIDER QUEEN

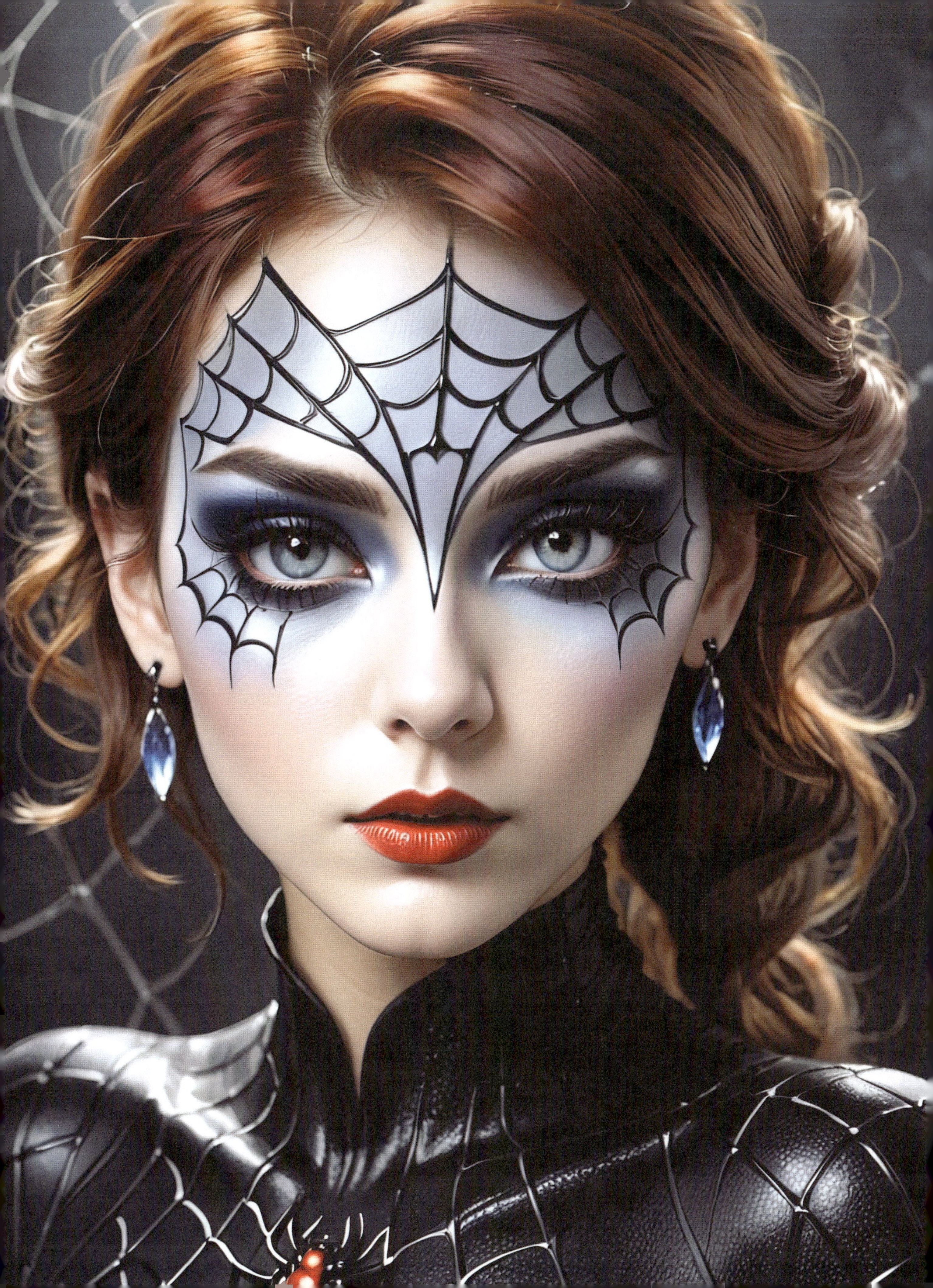

"IRIS ENCHANTRESS"

STEP-BY-STEP INSTRUCTIONS:

1. SKIN PREPARATION:

TOOLS: LIGHT FOUNDATION, SETTING POWDER.

INSTRUCTIONS: START BY APPLYING A LIGHT FOUNDATION EVENLY ACROSS THE FACE AND NECK TO CREATE A SMOOTH BASE. SET THE FOUNDATION WITH A TRANSLUCENT SETTING POWDER TO PREVENT ANY SHINE AND TO ENSURE THE MAKEUP STAYS IN PLACE.

2. EYES:

TOOLS: PURPLE EYESHADOW, SILVER EYESHADOW, BLACK EYELINER, MASCARA, FALSE EYELASHES (OPTIONAL).

INSTRUCTIONS: APPLY A RICH PURPLE EYESHADOW OVER THE EYELIDS, BLENDING UPWARDS TOWARDS THE BROW BONE. ADD SILVER EYESHADOW TO THE INNER CORNERS OF THE EYES TO BRIGHTEN THEM AND ADD A TOUCH OF SHIMMER. USE BLACK EYELINER TO DEFINE THE UPPER LASH LINE AND CREATE A SUBTLE WING AT THE OUTER CORNERS. APPLY MASCARA TO THE UPPER AND LOWER LASHES, AND ADD FALSE EYELASHES FOR EXTRA DRAMA IF DESIRED.

3. FACE DETAILING:

TOOLS: SILVER AND BLACK FACE PAINT, FINE BRUSHES, VIOLET HIGHLIGHTER.

INSTRUCTIONS: USING SILVER AND BLACK FACE PAINT, CREATE A SYMMETRICAL FLORAL PATTERN STARTING FROM THE TEMPLES AND EXTENDING TOWARDS THE FOREHEAD. ENSURE THE DESIGN IS ELEGANT AND FLOWING, INSPIRED BY THE SHAPES OF IRIS PETALS. HIGHLIGHT CERTAIN AREAS OF THE DESIGN WITH A VIOLET HIGHLIGHTER TO ADD DIMENSION AND A SOFT GLOW.

4. LIPS:

TOOLS: DEEP PURPLE LIPSTICK.

INSTRUCTIONS: APPLY A DEEP PURPLE LIPSTICK, ENSURING THE EDGES ARE PRECISE FOR A CLEAN FINISH. THE BOLD LIP COLOR COMPLEMENTS THE EYE MAKEUP AND TIES THE ENTIRE LOOK TOGETHER.

5. HAIR AND ACCESSORIES:

TOOLS: IRIS FLOWERS (REAL OR ARTIFICIAL), HAIRPINS, BLACK VEIL, ORNATE EARRINGS.

INSTRUCTIONS: STYLE THE HAIR IN LOOSE WAVES, PINNING IT BACK SLIGHTLY ON BOTH SIDES WITH IRIS FLOWERS. ATTACH A BLACK VEIL AT THE BACK OF THE HAIR, LETTING IT DRAPE ELEGANTLY OVER THE SHOULDERS. FINISH WITH ORNATE EARRINGS THAT ECHO THE BLACK AND GOLD DETAILS OF THE COSTUME.

6. COSTUME:

TOOLS: BLACK AND SILVER EMBROIDERED GOWN, GEMSTONE NECKLACE.

INSTRUCTIONS: DRESS IN AN ELABORATE BLACK AND SILVER EMBROIDERED GOWN THAT MATCHES THE INTRICATE MAKEUP DESIGN. ADD A GEMSTONE NECKLACE WITH A CENTRAL PIECE THAT DRAWS ATTENTION TO THE NECKLINE AND ENHANCES THE OVERALL REGAL APPEARANCE.

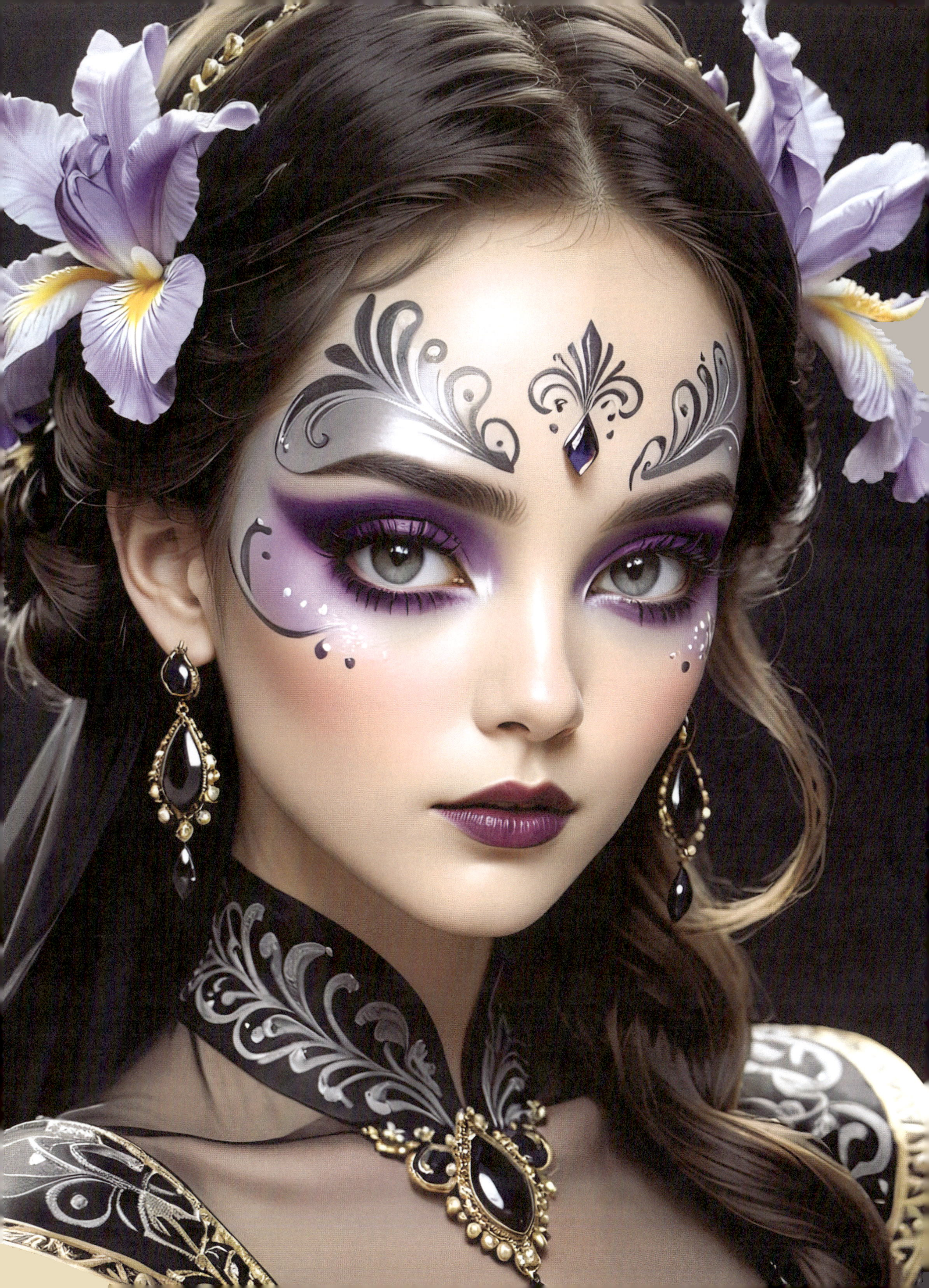

"Skeletal Specter"

Step-by-step instructions:

1. Skin Preparation:

Tools: Light foundation, setting powder.

Instructions: Begin by applying a light foundation to create a smooth, even base. Set the foundation with a translucent setting powder to ensure the makeup stays in place.

2. Face Detailing:

Tools: Black and white face paint, fine brushes.

Instructions: Start by using white face paint to cover the entire face and neck, creating the base for the skull effect. Then, with black face paint, carefully outline the skull design, focusing on the eye sockets, nose, and jawline. Add the intricate details, such as the teeth and cracks, to enhance the realism of the skull.

3. Eyes:

Tools: Black eyeliner, black eyeshadow, mascara.

Instructions: Use black eyeliner to outline the eye sockets, filling them in with black eyeshadow to deepen the hollowed effect. Apply mascara to the lashes to define the eyes, creating a stark contrast against the dark sockets.

4. Lips:

Tools: Black face paint, fine brush.

Instructions: Use black face paint to outline and fill in the lips, extending the lines outward to create a skeletal teeth effect. Ensure the teeth lines are sharp and evenly spaced for a striking appearance.

5. Neck and Chest Detailing:

Tools: Black and white body paint, fine brushes.

Instructions: Extend the skeletal design down the neck and chest using black and white body paint. Carefully paint the collarbones, ribs, and spine to create a realistic skeletal appearance. Ensure the lines are precise and symmetrical to maintain the illusion of exposed bones.

6. Accessories:

Tools: Antique-style earrings.

Instructions: Add a pair of antique-style earrings to complement the haunting, elegant look.

7. Costume:

Tools: Black gown or robe.

Instructions: Wear a flowing black gown or robe that matches the dark, eerie theme of the makeup. This will keep the focus on the skeletal design, emphasizing the ethereal and ghostly appearance.

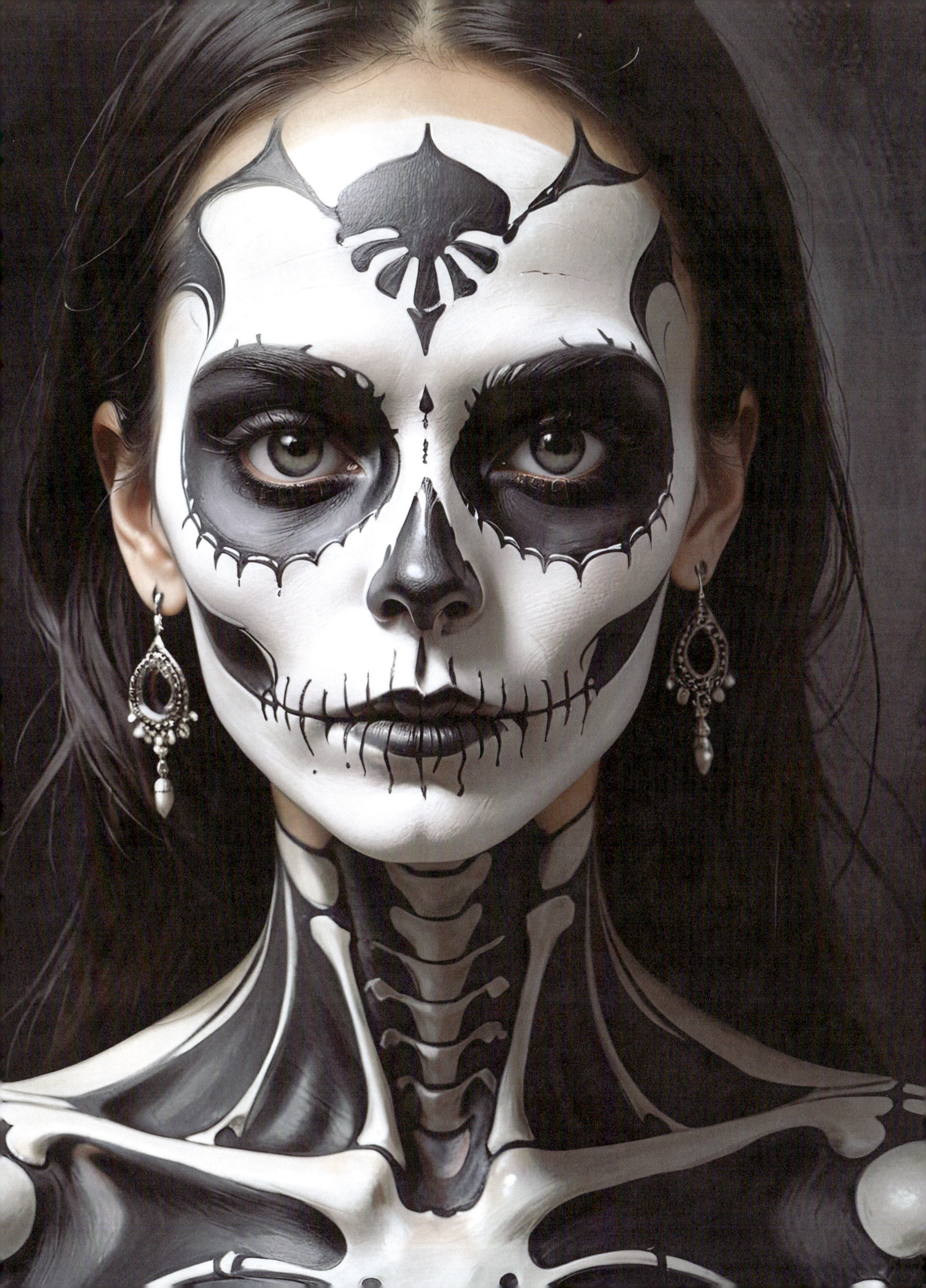

"PIRATE QUEEN"

STEP-BY-STEP INSTRUCTIONS:

1. SKIN PREPARATION:

TOOLS: PRIMER, FOUNDATION, SETTING POWDER.

INSTRUCTIONS: APPLY A PRIMER, THEN A MEDIUM COVERAGE FOUNDATION TO EVEN OUT THE SKIN TONE. SET WITH TRANSLUCENT POWDER.

2. FACE DETAILING:

TOOLS: BLACK FACE PAINT, FINE BRUSH.

INSTRUCTIONS: PAINT A BLACK MASK AROUND THE EYES WITH DETAILED EDGES. ADD A SKULL AND CROSSBONES SYMBOL ON THE FOREHEAD.

3. EYES:

TOOLS: BLACK EYELINER, DARK EYESHADOW, MASCARA.

INSTRUCTIONS: LINE THE EYES WITH BLACK EYELINER, USE DARK EYESHADOW TO ADD DEPTH, AND APPLY MASCARA FOR DEFINED LASHES.

4. LIPS:

TOOLS: NUDE LIPSTICK.

INSTRUCTIONS: APPLY A NUDE LIPSTICK TO KEEP THE FOCUS ON THE EYES AND FACE DETAILING.

5. HAIR:

TOOLS: HAIR TIES, SEA SALT SPRAY.

INSTRUCTIONS: CREATE TWO LOOSE BRAIDS AND USE SEA SALT SPRAY FOR A TOUSLED, TEXTURED LOOK.

6. ACCESSORIES & COSTUME:

TOOLS: PIRATE HAT, GOLD HOOP EARRINGS, PIRATE COSTUME.

INSTRUCTIONS: COMPLETE THE LOOK WITH A PIRATE HAT, GOLD HOOP EARRINGS, AND A DARK, RUGGED PIRATE COSTUME.

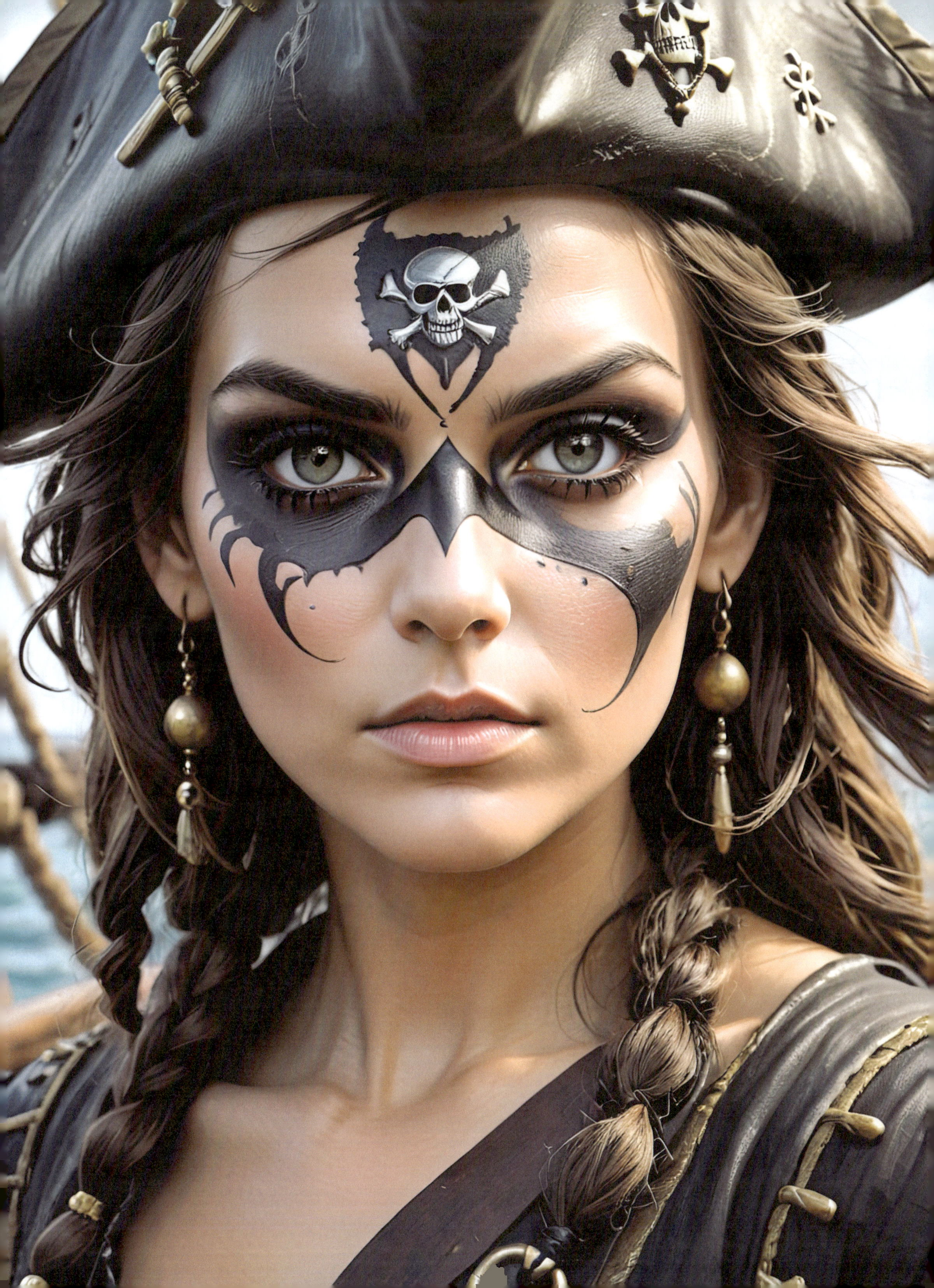

STEP-BY-STEP INSTRUCTIONS:

1. SKIN PREPARATION:

TOOLS: PRIMER, FOUNDATION, BRONZER, HIGHLIGHTER.

INSTRUCTIONS: BEGIN WITH A PRIMER FOR SMOOTH APPLICATION, APPLY A WARM-TONED FOUNDATION TO CREATE A FLAWLESS BASE, AND USE BRONZER TO CONTOUR THE CHEEKS. ADD A SUBTLE HIGHLIGHTER TO THE HIGH POINTS OF THE FACE FOR A GLOWING EFFECT.

2. EYES:

TOOLS: GOLD EYESHADOW, BLACK LIQUID EYELINER, MASCARA.

INSTRUCTIONS: APPLY GOLD EYESHADOW OVER THE EYELIDS, THEN USE BLACK LIQUID EYELINER TO CREATE AN EXAGGERATED CAT-EYE LOOK, EXTENDING THE LINER TOWARD THE TEMPLES. FINISH WITH MASCARA FOR VOLUMINOUS LASHES.

3. FACE DETAILING:

TOOLS: BLACK FACE PAINT, FINE BRUSH, GOLD FACE PAINT.

INSTRUCTIONS: USE BLACK FACE PAINT TO DRAW HORIZONTAL LINES ACROSS THE FOREHEAD, NOSE BRIDGE, AND CHEEKS. HIGHLIGHT THE DESIGNS WITH GOLD FACE PAINT FOR AN INTRICATE AND ROYAL LOOK.

3. LIPS:

TOOLS: NUDE LIPSTICK OR CLEAR GLOSS.

INSTRUCTIONS: KEEP THE LIPS NEUTRAL WITH A NUDE LIPSTICK OR A TOUCH OF CLEAR GLOSS TO ENSURE THE FOCUS REMAINS ON THE EYES AND FACE DETAILING.

5. HAIR & HEADPIECE:

TOOLS: EGYPTIAN-STYLE HEADDRESS.

INSTRUCTIONS: SECURE HAIR IN A SLEEK STYLE AND PLACE THE TRADITIONAL EGYPTIAN HEADDRESS SECURELY ON THE HEAD.

6. ACCESSORIES & COSTUME:

TOOLS: GOLD STATEMENT NECKLACE, GOLD EARRINGS, EGYPTIAN-STYLE DRESS.

INSTRUCTIONS: ADD A BOLD GOLD NECKLACE, STATEMENT EARRINGS, AND COMPLETE THE ENSEMBLE WITH A TRADITIONAL EGYPTIAN-STYLE DRESS FOR AN AUTHENTIC QUEEN OF THE NILE APPEARANCE.

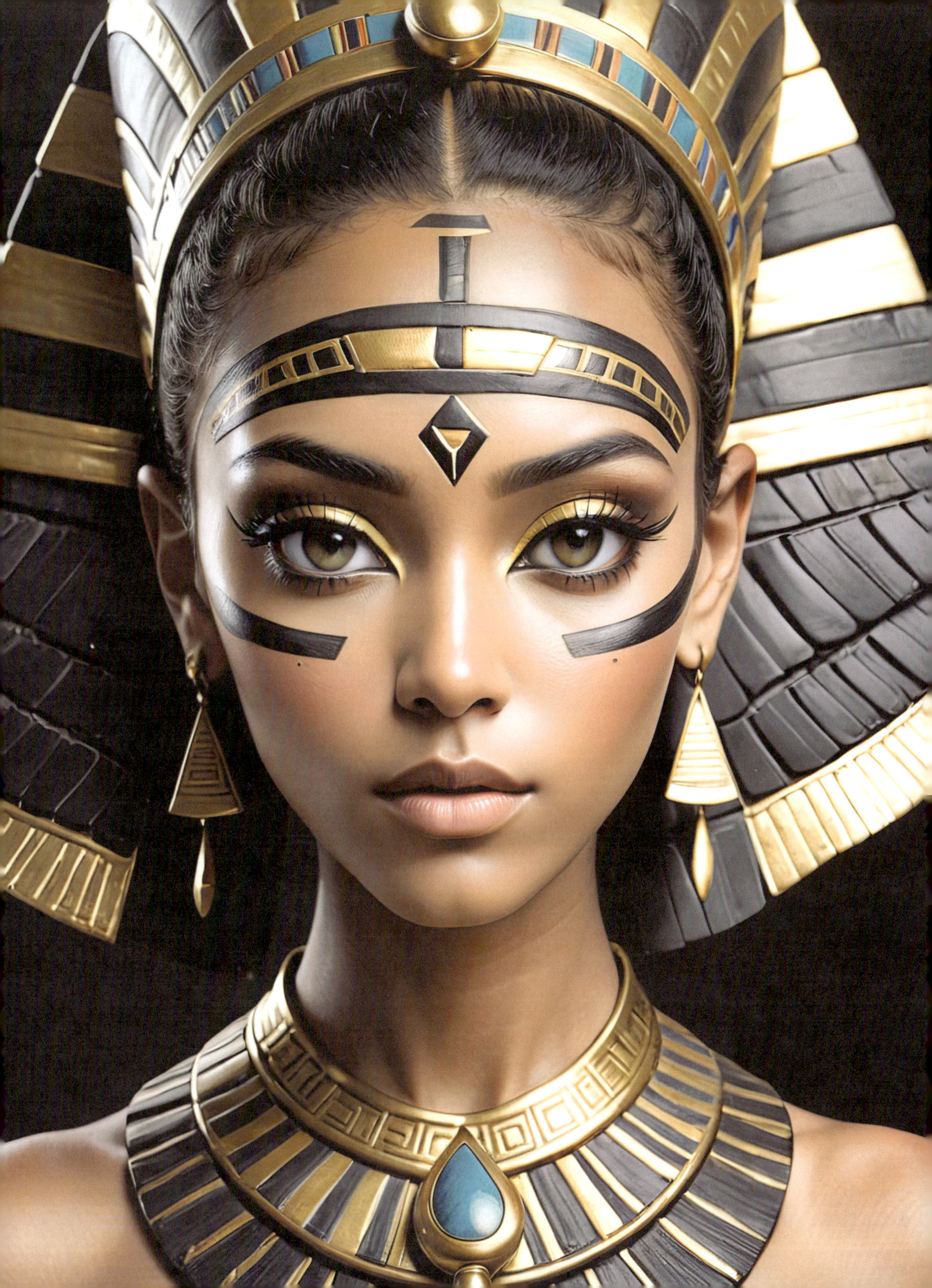

"WESTERN PHANTOM"

STEP-BY-STEP INSTRUCTIONS:

1. SKIN PREPARATION:

TOOLS: PRIMER, FULL COVERAGE FOUNDATION, SETTING POWDER.

INSTRUCTIONS: BEGIN WITH A PRIMER TO CREATE A SMOOTH BASE. APPLY A FULL COVERAGE FOUNDATION TO ACHIEVE A FLAWLESS, EVEN COMPLEXION. SET THE FOUNDATION WITH A SETTING POWDER TO ENSURE A MATTE FINISH.

2. EYES:

TOOLS: BLACK EYESHADOW, BLENDING BRUSH, BLACK EYELINER.

INSTRUCTIONS: APPLY BLACK EYESHADOW TO THE EYELIDS, BLENDING IT OUTWARD TO CREATE A SMOKY EFFECT. USE BLACK EYELINER TO LINE THE UPPER AND LOWER LASH LINES, EXTENDING SLIGHTLY BEYOND THE OUTER CORNERS FOR A MORE INTENSE LOOK.

3. FACE DETAILING:

TOOLS: BLACK AND WHITE FACE PAINT, FINE BRUSHES.

INSTRUCTIONS: USE WHITE FACE PAINT TO CREATE A GHOSTLY BASE. APPLY BLACK FACE PAINT TO DRAW SHARP, THORN-LIKE PATTERNS AROUND THE EYES, EXTENDING TOWARDS THE FOREHEAD AND CHEEKS. ADD ADDITIONAL BLACK DETAILING ALONG THE NOSE AND JAWLINE FOR A DRAMATIC CONTRAST.

4. LIPS:

TOOLS: DEEP RED OR BLACK LIPSTICK.

INSTRUCTIONS: APPLY A DEEP RED OR BLACK LIPSTICK TO THE LIPS, CREATING A BOLD, DEFINED SHAPE.

5. HAIR & HEADPIECE:

TOOLS: COWBOY HAT, HAIR GEL OR WAX.

INSTRUCTIONS: STYLE THE HAIR BACK OR IN A LOW PONYTAIL, USING HAIR GEL OR WAX FOR A SLEEK LOOK. PLACE A RUGGED COWBOY HAT ON THE HEAD TO COMPLETE THE WESTERN AESTHETIC.

6. ACCESSORIES & COSTUME:

TOOLS: LEATHER JACKET, BANDANA, SILVER ACCESSORIES.

INSTRUCTIONS: PAIR THE LOOK WITH A WORN LEATHER JACKET, A BANDANA AROUND THE NECK, AND SILVER ACCESSORIES LIKE EARRINGS OR A BOLO TIE TO EMBODY THE SPIRIT OF A HAUNTED WESTERN GUNSLINGER.

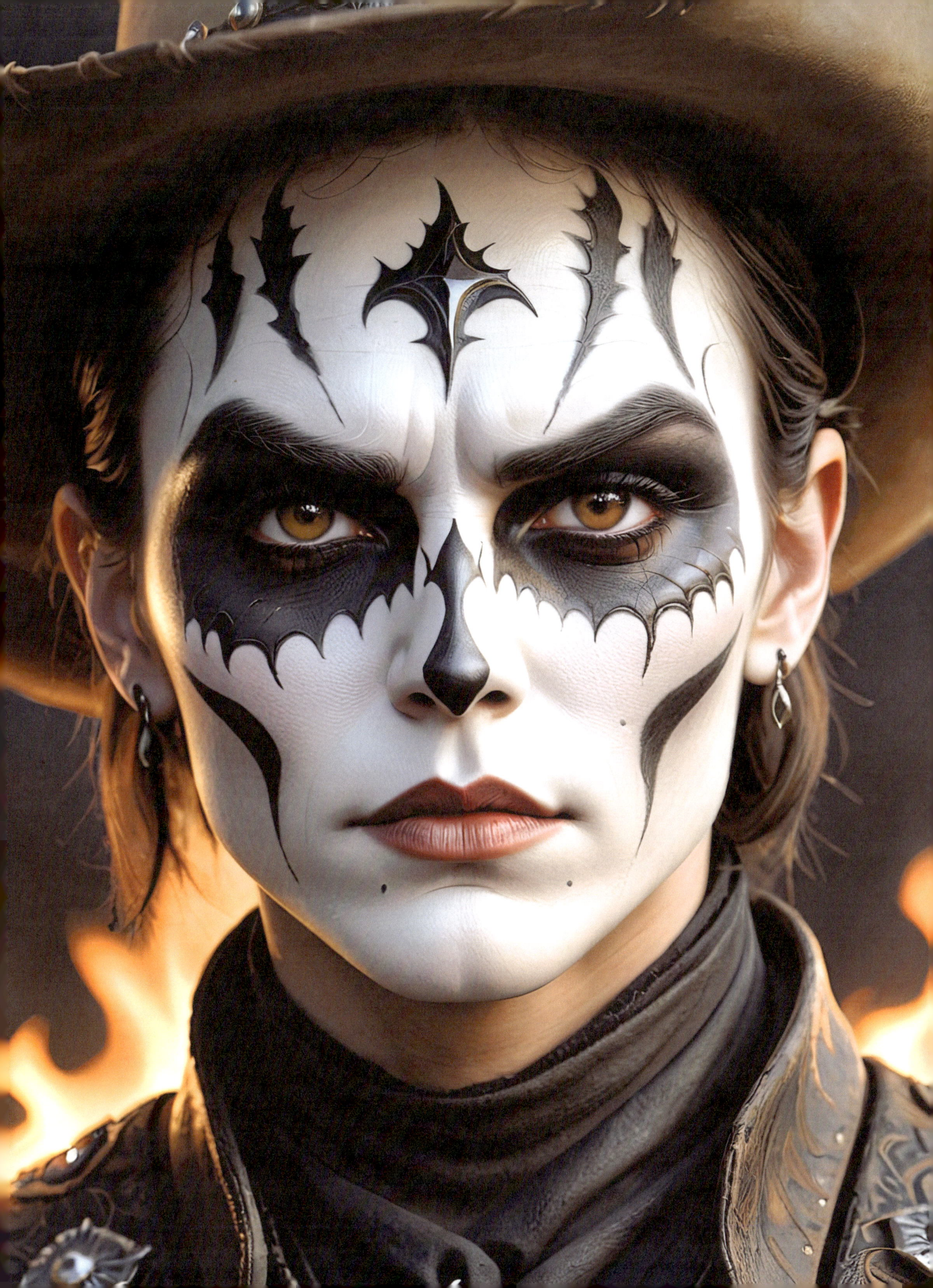

"ELEGANT CLOWN"

STEP-BY-STEP INSTRUCTIONS:

1. SKIN PREPARATION:

TOOLS: PRIMER, WHITE FACE PAINT OR FOUNDATION, SETTING POWDER.

INSTRUCTIONS: START BY APPLYING A PRIMER TO CREATE A SMOOTH SURFACE. USE A WHITE FACE PAINT OR FOUNDATION TO COVER THE ENTIRE FACE, ENSURING AN EVEN APPLICATION. SET WITH A TRANSLUCENT SETTING POWDER TO LOCK IN THE MAKEUP.

2. EYES:

TOOLS: BLUE EYESHADOW, BLACK EYELINER, MASCARA.

INSTRUCTIONS: APPLY A VIBRANT BLUE EYESHADOW OVER THE EYELIDS, EXTENDING SLIGHTLY BEYOND THE CREASE FOR A DRAMATIC EFFECT. USE BLACK EYELINER TO DEFINE THE EYES, CREATING A SHARP LINE ALONG THE UPPER AND LOWER LASH LINES. FINISH WITH A COAT OF MASCARA TO ENHANCE THE LASHES.

3. FACE DETAILING:

TOOLS: BLACK AND WHITE FACE PAINT, FINE BRUSH.

INSTRUCTIONS: USE BLACK FACE PAINT TO CREATE SYMMETRICAL DIAMOND SHAPES ABOVE AND BELOW THE EYES, EXTENDING FROM THE EYEBROWS TO THE CHEEKS. DRAW A BLACK, NARROW LINE FROM THE TIP OF THE NOSE TO THE UPPER LIP, MIMICKING A TRADITIONAL CLOWN LOOK. ADD SMALL BLACK DOTS ABOVE THE EYEBROWS AND ON THE CHEEKS FOR ADDED DETAIL.

4. LIPS:

TOOLS: BLACK LIPSTICK.

INSTRUCTIONS: APPLY BLACK LIPSTICK TO THE LIPS, ENSURING A CLEAN AND PRECISE OUTLINE. THE LIPS SHOULD BE DEFINED BUT NOT OVERLY EXAGGERATED, MAINTAINING THE ELEGANT ASPECT OF THE LOOK.

5. HAIR & HEADPIECE:

TOOLS: WIG OR HAIR ACCESSORIES, LARGE BOW OR HEADPIECE.

INSTRUCTIONS: STYLE THE HAIR IN TIGHT CURLS OR USE A WIG TO ACHIEVE THE DESIRED LOOK. ADD A LARGE, DECORATIVE BOW OR HEADPIECE IN BLUE AND BLACK TO MATCH THE OVERALL COLOR SCHEME, SECURING IT FIRMLY ON THE TOP OF THE HEAD.

6. COSTUME & ACCESSORIES:

TOOLS: CLOWN COLLAR, MATCHING EARRINGS, AND NECKLACE.

INSTRUCTIONS: WEAR A RUFFLED CLOWN COLLAR IN A MATCHING BLUE AND WHITE COLOR SCHEME. PAIR THE LOOK WITH BOLD EARRINGS AND A STATEMENT NECKLACE FEATURING RED AND BLACK GEMSTONES TO ADD A TOUCH OF SOPHISTICATION. THE COSTUME SHOULD BE ELEGANT AND COORDINATED, COMPLEMENTING THE MAKEUP FOR A POLISHED FINISH.

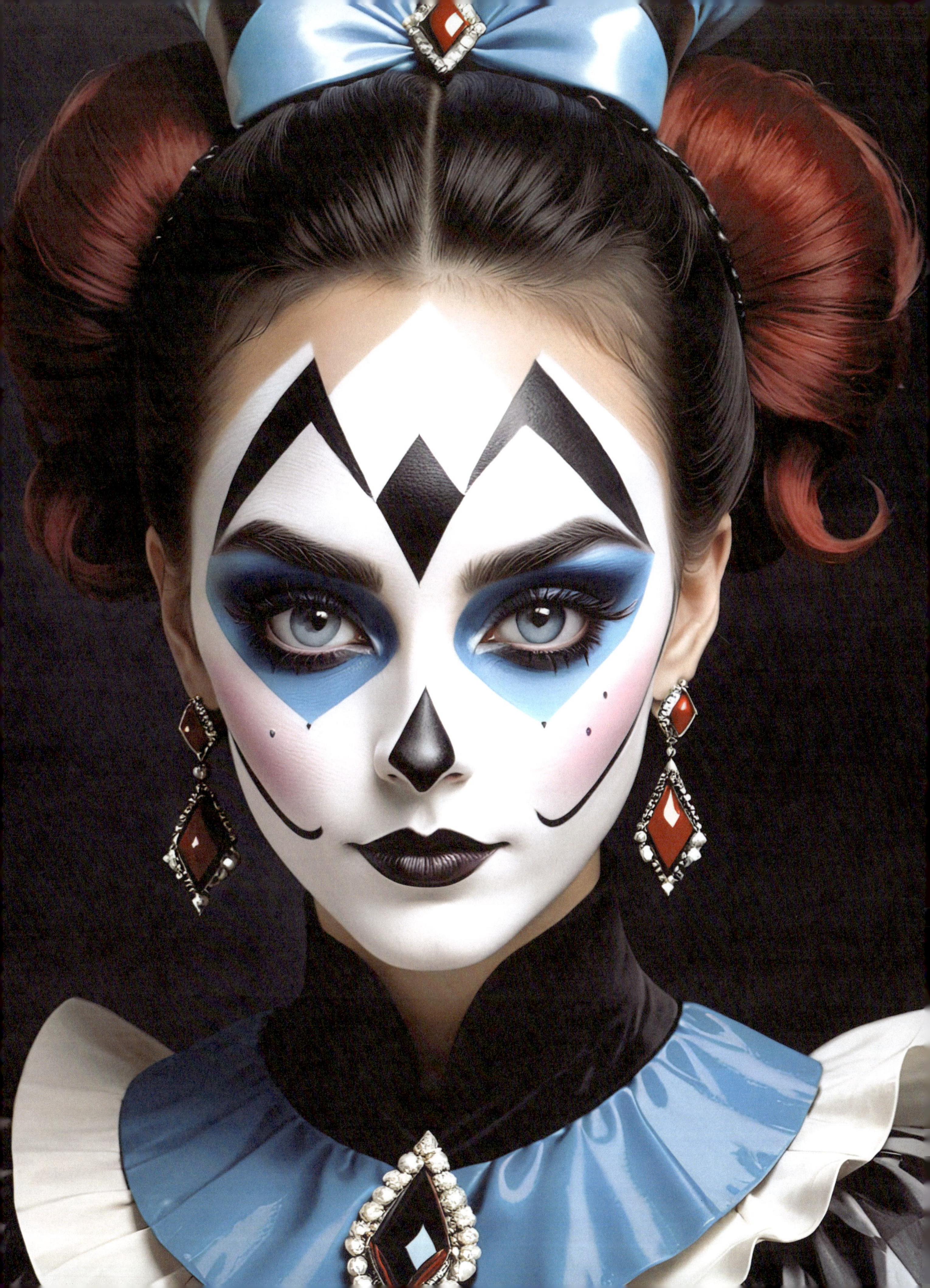

"ETHEREAL GOTHIC BRIDE"

STEP-BY-STEP INSTRUCTIONS:

1. SKIN PREPARATION:

TOOLS: PRIMER, PALE WHITE FOUNDATION, SETTING POWDER.

INSTRUCTIONS: BEGIN BY APPLYING A PRIMER TO CREATE A SMOOTH BASE. USE A PALE WHITE FOUNDATION TO ACHIEVE AN ETHEREAL, GHOSTLY LOOK, COVERING THE ENTIRE FACE AND NECK. SET THE FOUNDATION WITH A TRANSLUCENT SETTING POWDER TO ENSURE A MATTE FINISH.

2. EYES:

TOOLS: BLACK AND GRAY EYESHADOW, EYELINER, MASCARA.

INSTRUCTIONS: APPLY A DARK GRAY EYESHADOW OVER THE EYELIDS, EXTENDING IT SLIGHTLY ABOVE THE CREASE. BLEND BLACK EYESHADOW INTO THE OUTER CORNERS AND LOWER LASH LINE FOR A SMOKY EFFECT. USE BLACK EYELINER TO DEFINE THE EYES, KEEPING THE LINE CLOSE TO THE LASHES. APPLY MASCARA TO ENHANCE THE LASHES, GIVING THEM A DRAMATIC LIFT.

3. FACE DETAILING:

TOOLS: BLACK FACE PAINT, FINE BRUSH.

INSTRUCTIONS: CREATE A TEAR-LIKE BLACK DROPLET DESIGN ON THE CENTER OF THE FOREHEAD USING BLACK FACE PAINT. ADD SIMILAR DESIGNS UNDER THE EYES, MIMICKING THE APPEARANCE OF GOTHIC-STYLE TEARS. DRAW DELICATE BLACK SPIKES RADIATING FROM THE OUTER EDGES OF THE EYES FOR A HAUNTING EFFECT.

4. LIPS:

TOOLS: BLACK LIPSTICK.

INSTRUCTIONS: APPLY BLACK LIPSTICK TO THE LIPS, FOCUSING ON ACHIEVING A SHARP, DEFINED OUTLINE. THE LIPS SHOULD CONTRAST STARKLY WITH THE PALE SKIN, ENHANCING THE GOTHIC THEME.

5. HAIR & VEIL:

TOOLS: BLACK OR DARK HAIR ACCESSORIES, SHEER BLACK VEIL.

INSTRUCTIONS: STYLE THE HAIR IN LOOSE WAVES OR TUCK IT UNDER A BLACK HEADBAND. ATTACH A SHEER BLACK VEIL ADORNED WITH DARK FLOWERS OR LACE TO COMPLETE THE BRIDAL LOOK, SECURING IT AT THE BACK OF THE HEAD.

6. COSTUME & ACCESSORIES:

TOOLS: GOTHIC LACE CHOKER, BLACK EARRINGS.

INSTRUCTIONS: WEAR A GOTHIC LACE CHOKER TO ACCENTUATE THE NECK AND A PAIR OF BLACK OR DARK GEMSTONE EARRINGS FOR A TOUCH OF ELEGANCE. THE COSTUME SHOULD CONSIST OF DARK, FLOWING FABRICS, WITH LACE DETAILING TO COMPLEMENT THE OVERALL GOTHIC BRIDAL THEME.

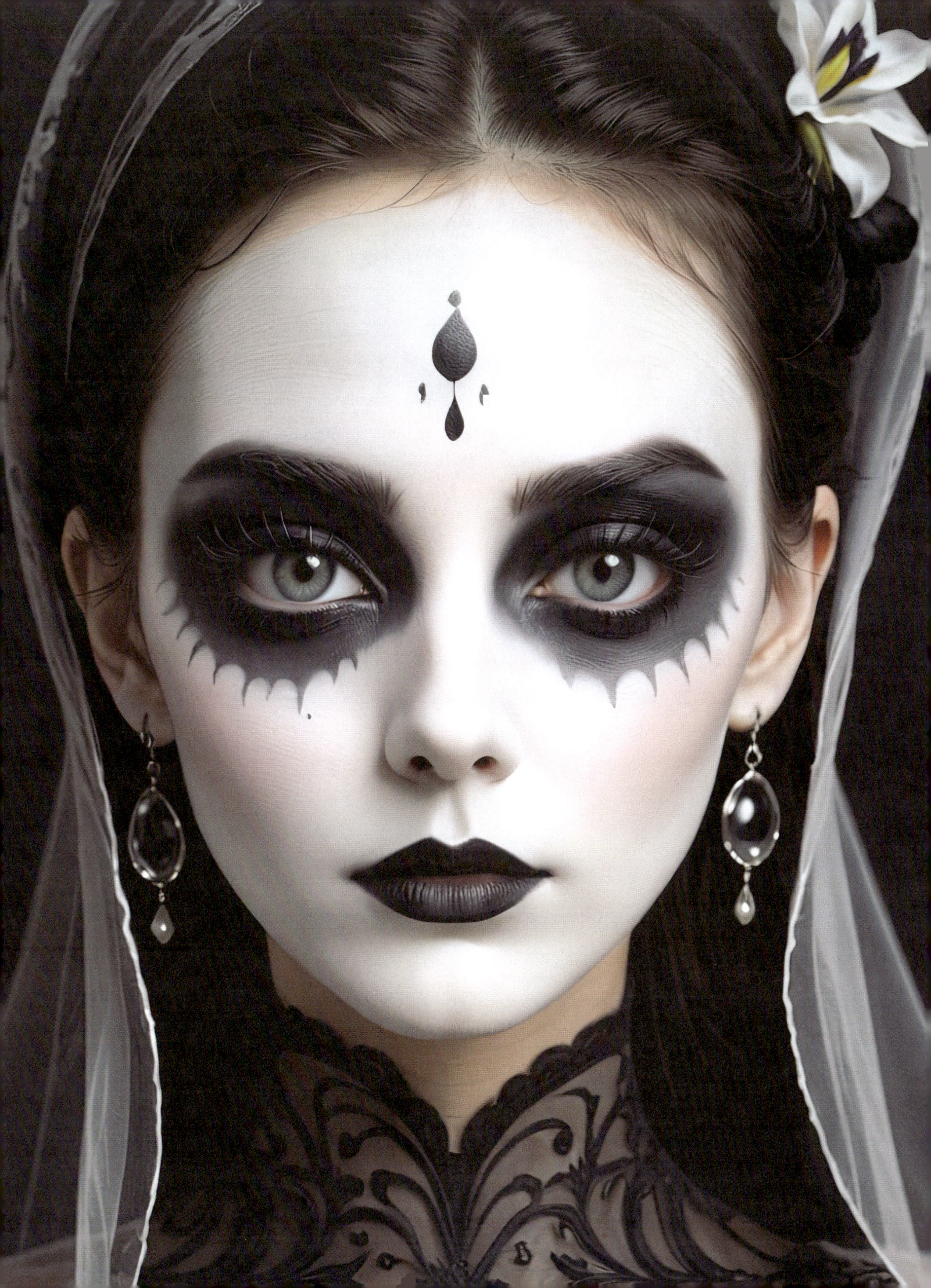

"SAMURAI WARRIOR MAKEUP"

STEP-BY-STEP INSTRUCTIONS:

1. SKIN PREPARATION:

TOOLS: PRIMER, WHITE FACE PAINT, SETTING POWDER.

INSTRUCTIONS: START BY APPLYING A PRIMER TO ENSURE SMOOTH APPLICATION AND LONG-LASTING MAKEUP. USE WHITE FACE PAINT TO COVER THE ENTIRE FACE, CREATING A FLAWLESS BASE. SET THE PAINT WITH A TRANSLUCENT SETTING POWDER TO PREVENT SMUDGING.

2. EYES:

TOOLS: RED AND BLACK EYESHADOW, EYELINER, MASCARA.

INSTRUCTIONS: APPLY A RED EYESHADOW AROUND THE EYES, FOCUSING ON THE EYELIDS AND EXTENDING OUTWARD INTO A SHARP, WINGED SHAPE. ADD BLACK EYESHADOW TO DEFINE THE CREASE AND OUTER CORNERS OF THE EYES, BLENDING SLIGHTLY INTO THE RED. USE BLACK EYELINER TO CREATE A DRAMATIC WING, ENHANCING THE SHAPE OF THE EYES. FINISH WITH A COAT OF MASCARA TO DEFINE THE LASHES.

3. FACE DETAILING:

TOOLS: BLACK AND RED FACE PAINT, FINE BRUSH.

INSTRUCTIONS: USE BLACK FACE PAINT TO CREATE BOLD, GRAPHIC DESIGNS ON THE FOREHEAD AND CHEEKS, RESEMBLING TRADITIONAL SAMURAI WARRIOR MASKS. INCORPORATE RED ACCENTS WITHIN THE BLACK DESIGNS TO ADD DEPTH AND INTENSITY. ENSURE THE LINES ARE CLEAN AND PRECISE FOR A SHARP, FIERCE LOOK.

4. LIPS:

TOOLS: RED LIPSTICK.

INSTRUCTIONS: APPLY A VIBRANT RED LIPSTICK TO THE LIPS, KEEPING THE EDGES CRISP AND DEFINED. THE BOLD RED LIPS SHOULD COMPLEMENT THE RED ACCENTS IN THE EYE MAKEUP AND FACE DETAILING.

5. HAIR & ACCESSORIES:

TOOLS: HAIR GEL, TRADITIONAL SAMURAI HAIR ACCESSORIES (E.G., HAIRPINS, TASSELS).

INSTRUCTIONS: STYLE THE HAIR INTO A SLEEK BUN OR PONYTAIL, USING HAIR GEL TO SMOOTH ANY FLYAWAYS. ADD TRADITIONAL SAMURAI HAIR ACCESSORIES, SUCH AS HAIRPINS OR TASSELS, TO ENHANCE THE OVERALL LOOK. THE ACCESSORIES SHOULD BE POSITIONED TO FRAME THE FACE, COMPLEMENTING THE MAKEUP.

6. COSTUME & ARMOR:

TOOLS: SAMURAI ARMOR OR COSTUME, RED AND BLACK FABRIC ACCENTS.

INSTRUCTIONS: WEAR A SAMURAI-INSPIRED COSTUME WITH ARMOR DETAILING TO COMPLETE THE LOOK. INCORPORATE RED AND BLACK FABRIC ACCENTS THAT TIE INTO THE MAKEUP DESIGN. THE COSTUME SHOULD REFLECT THE STRENGTH AND HONOR OF A SAMURAI WARRIOR, WITH ATTENTION TO HISTORICAL ACCURACY IN THE CHOICE OF MATERIALS AND PATTERNS.

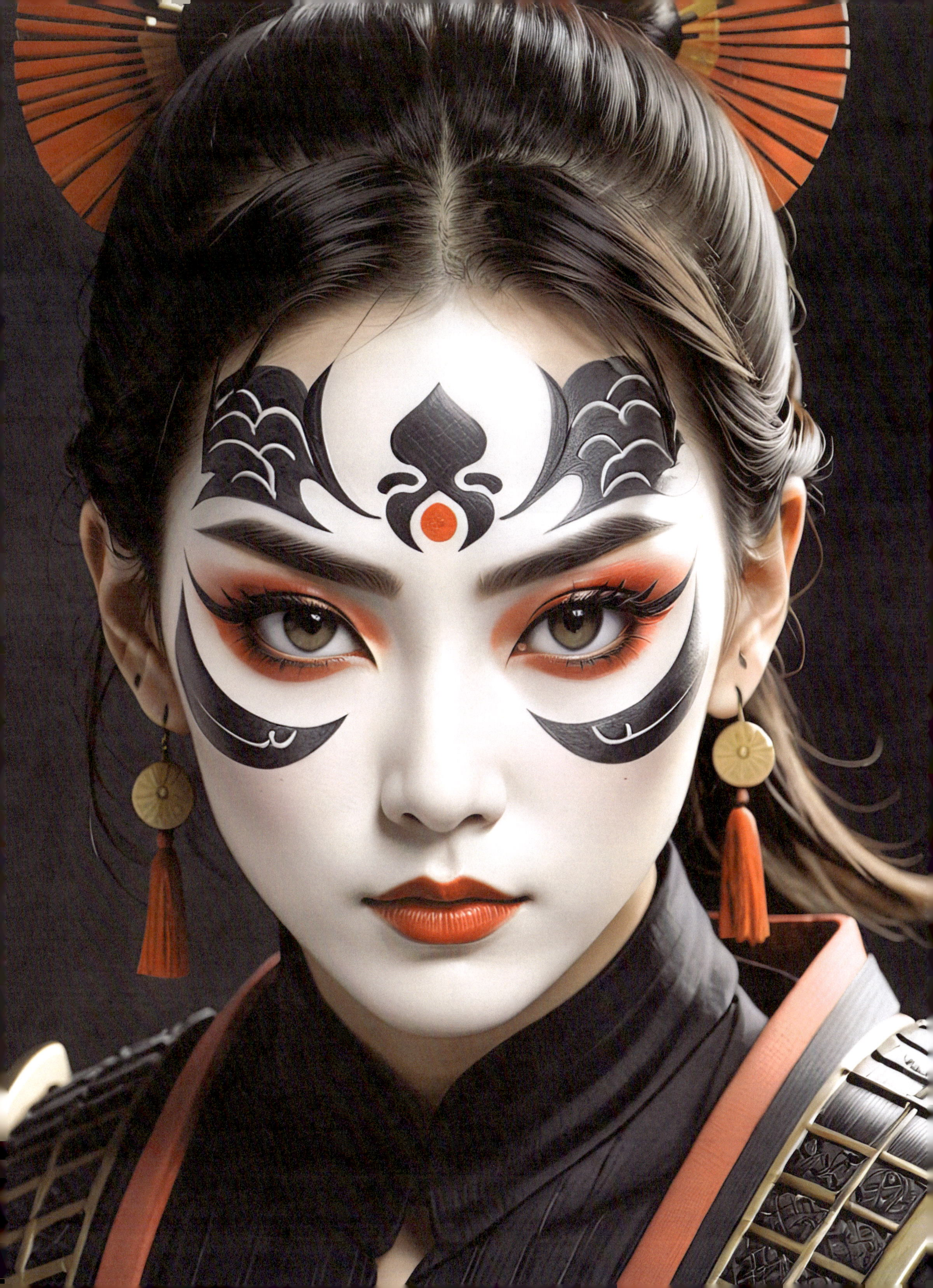

"DARK WITCH"

STEP-BY-STEP INSTRUCTIONS:

SKIN PREPARATION:

TOOLS: PRIMER, LIGHT FOUNDATION, TRANSLUCENT POWDER.

INSTRUCTIONS: APPLY PRIMER TO CREATE A SMOOTH BASE AND ENSURE LONG-LASTING MAKEUP. USE A LIGHT FOUNDATION TO ACHIEVE A PALE, ALMOST PORCELAIN-LIKE COMPLEXION. SET THE FOUNDATION WITH A TRANSLUCENT POWDER TO PREVENT SHINE AND ENSURE THE MAKEUP STAYS IN PLACE.

EYES:

TOOLS: PURPLE AND BLACK EYESHADOW, EYELINER, FALSE EYELASHES, MASCARA.

INSTRUCTIONS: APPLY PURPLE EYESHADOW ACROSS THE ENTIRE EYELID, BLENDING IT UP TOWARDS THE BROW BONE TO CREATE A DEEP, DRAMATIC EFFECT. USE BLACK EYESHADOW ON THE OUTER CORNERS OF THE EYES, BLENDING IT INTO THE PURPLE FOR A SEAMLESS TRANSITION. APPLY EYELINER TO CREATE A PRECISE, ELONGATED WING ALONG THE LASH LINE. FINISH BY APPLYING FALSE EYELASHES FOR ADDED INTENSITY, AND COAT WITH MASCARA TO DEFINE THE LASHES.

FACE DETAILING:

TOOLS: BLACK FACE PAINT, FINE BRUSH, GREEN CRYSTAL OR FOREHEAD STICKER.

INSTRUCTIONS: USE BLACK FACE PAINT TO DRAW MYSTICAL SYMBOLS OR DESIGNS ON THE FOREHEAD, CREATING A SYMMETRICAL PATTERN ON BOTH SIDES OF THE FACE. PLACE A GREEN CRYSTAL OR STICKER AT THE CENTER OF THE FOREHEAD TO ADD A MAGICAL, MYSTERIOUS TOUCH.

LIPS:

TOOLS: BLACK LIPSTICK, LIP LINER.

INSTRUCTIONS: OUTLINE THE LIPS WITH BLACK LIP LINER, CAREFULLY DEFINING THEIR SHAPE. FILL IN THE LIPS WITH BLACK LIPSTICK, ENSURING EVEN COVERAGE. THE BLACK LIPS WILL ADD A TOUCH OF DARK ELEGANCE TO THE OVERALL LOOK.

HAIR & ACCESSORIES:

TOOLS: WIG OR HAIR DYE (IF NEEDED), WITCH HAT, GREEN AND BLACK ACCESSORIES.

INSTRUCTIONS: STYLE THE HAIR IN WAVES FOR ADDED VOLUME, OR USE A WIG IF NECESSARY. ADD A WITCH HAT TO COMPLETE THE LOOK. CHOOSE JEWELRY IN GREEN AND BLACK TONES TO MATCH THE MAKEUP AND COSTUME, ENHANCING THE DARK, MAGICAL VIBE.

COSTUME:

TOOLS: WITCH COSTUME, BLACK LACE, GREEN ACCENTS.

INSTRUCTIONS: WEAR A GOTHIC-STYLE WITCH COSTUME, PREFERABLY WITH BLACK LACE AND GREEN DETAILS TO COMPLEMENT THE MAKEUP. THE COSTUME SHOULD BE ELEGANT YET MYSTERIOUS, REFLECTING THE DARK, MAGICAL CHARACTER OF THE OVERALL APPEARANCE.

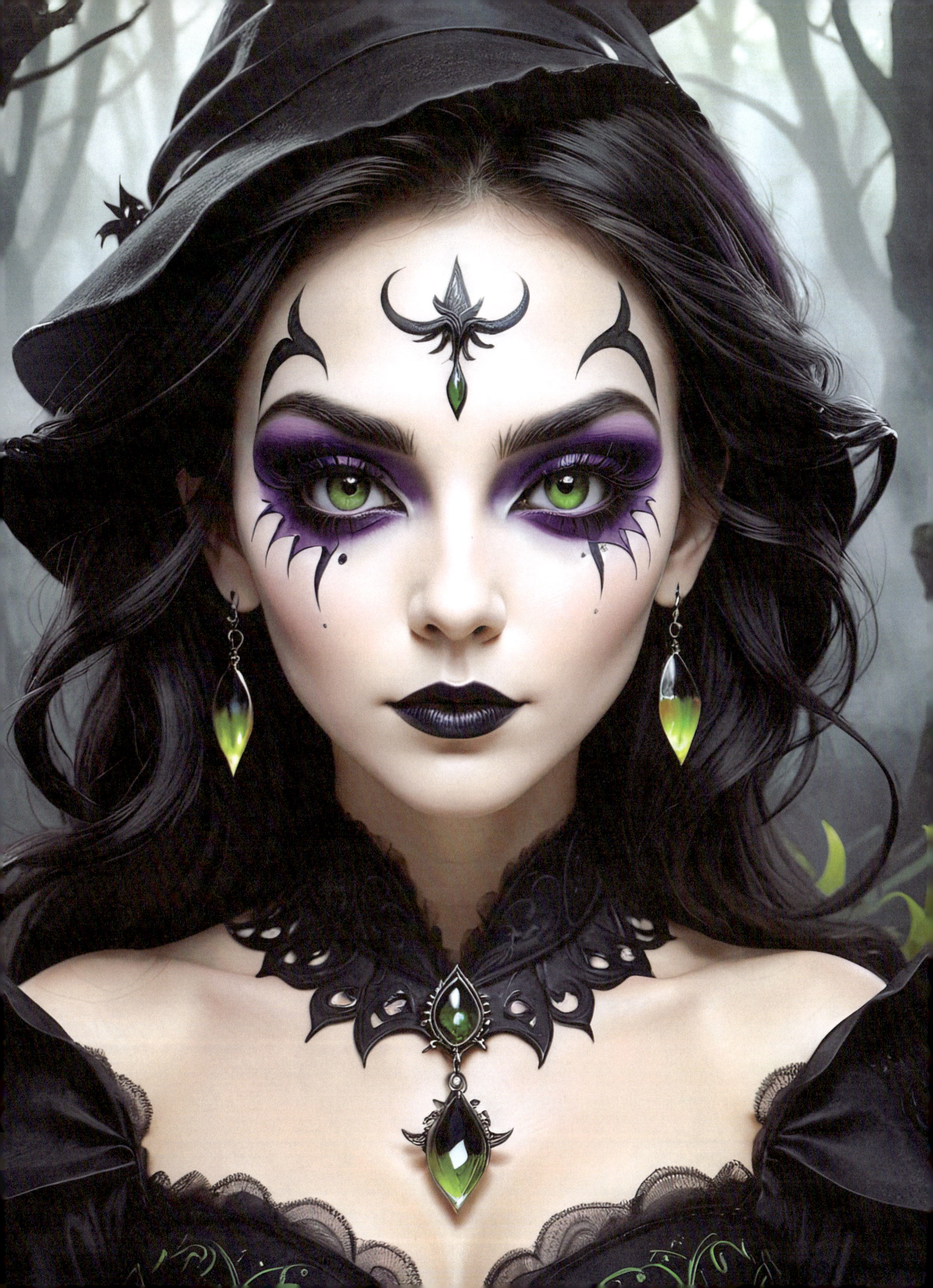

"INFERNAL DEMON"

STEP-BY-STEP INSTRUCTIONS:

SKIN PREPARATION:

TOOLS: PRIMER, WHITE FACE PAINT, TRANSLUCENT SETTING POWDER.

INSTRUCTIONS: START BY APPLYING A PRIMER TO ENSURE THE MAKEUP LASTS LONGER AND ADHERES SMOOTHLY. COVER THE ENTIRE FACE WITH WHITE FACE PAINT, CREATING A STARK, GHOSTLY BASE. SET THE PAINT WITH A TRANSLUCENT POWDER TO KEEP IT IN PLACE AND PREVENT SMUDGING.

EYES:

TOOLS: BLACK EYESHADOW, BLACK EYELINER, RED CONTACT LENSES, MASCARA.

INSTRUCTIONS: APPLY BLACK EYESHADOW AROUND THE EYES, EXTENDING IT OUTWARD INTO A SHARP, JAGGED PATTERN TO MIMIC THE LOOK OF CRACKED OR BURNING SKIN. USE BLACK EYELINER TO DEFINE THE EYES, CREATING A DRAMATIC, SMOLDERING EFFECT. ENHANCE THE LOOK WITH RED CONTACT LENSES TO GIVE THE EYES AN INTENSE, INFERNAL GLOW. FINISH WITH A LAYER OF MASCARA TO EMPHASIZE THE LASHES.

FACE DETAILING:

TOOLS: BLACK FACE PAINT, FINE BRUSH.

INSTRUCTIONS: USE BLACK FACE PAINT TO DRAW INTRICATE, SYMMETRICAL PATTERNS ON THE FOREHEAD AND AROUND THE EYES, MIMICKING DEMONIC OR SKELETAL DESIGNS. EXTEND THE DETAILING DOWN TO THE CHEEKS AND CHIN, USING SHARP, CLEAN LINES FOR A MENACING LOOK. ADD SUBTLE SHADING WITHIN THE BLACK AREAS TO CREATE DEPTH AND A MORE THREE-DIMENSIONAL EFFECT.

LIPS:

TOOLS: BLACK LIPSTICK, FINE BRUSH.

INSTRUCTIONS: APPLY BLACK LIPSTICK TO THE LIPS, KEEPING THE EDGES SHARP AND DEFINED. TO ADD TO THE DEMONIC APPEARANCE, USE A FINE BRUSH TO EXTEND THIN BLACK LINES FROM THE CORNERS OF THE MOUTH OUTWARD, MIMICKING THE LOOK OF A STITCHED OR SCARRED GRIN.

HORNS & ACCESSORIES:

TOOLS: DEMON HORNS (HEADBAND OR PROSTHETIC), BLACK HAIR DYE OR WIG, HAIR GEL.

INSTRUCTIONS: PLACE THE DEMON HORNS SECURELY ON THE HEAD, BLENDING THEM INTO THE HAIRLINE USING HAIR GEL OR PROSTHETIC ADHESIVE IF NEEDED. STYLE THE HAIR TO FLOW AROUND THE HORNS, USING A BLACK WIG OR HAIR DYE IF NECESSARY TO ACHIEVE THE DARK, SINISTER LOOK. ENSURE THE HORNS ARE POSITIONED SYMMETRICALLY AND ADD TO THE OVERALL DEMONIC AESTHETIC.

COSTUME:

TOOLS: GOTHIC OR DEMON-INSPIRED COSTUME, BLACK AND SILVER ACCENTS.

INSTRUCTIONS: WEAR A COSTUME THAT EMBODIES THE ESSENCE OF A POWERFUL DEMON, INCORPORATING GOTHIC ELEMENTS AND DARK, INTRICATE DESIGNS. LOOK FOR BLACK AND SILVER ACCENTS THAT MATCH THE MAKEUP, SUCH AS DETAILED ARMOR OR ROBES WITH MENACING PATTERNS. THE COSTUME SHOULD ENHANCE THE OVERALL INFERNAL APPEARANCE, MAKING THE CHARACTER LOOK BOTH TERRIFYING AND FORMIDABLE.

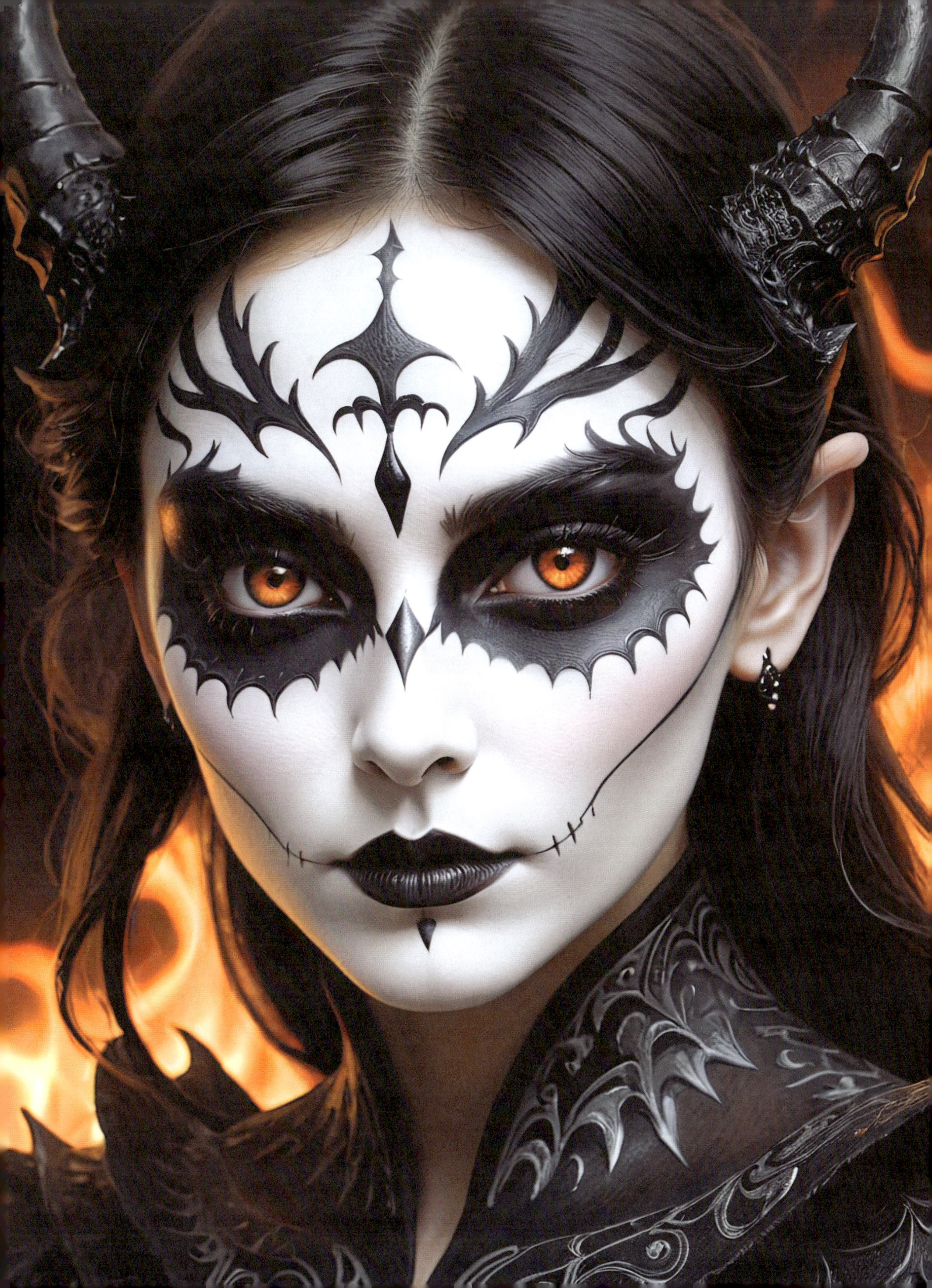

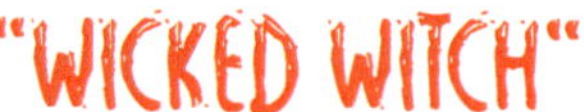

"WICKED WITCH"

STEP-BY-STEP INSTRUCTIONS:

SKIN PREPARATION:

TOOLS: PRIMER, GREEN FACE PAINT, TRANSLUCENT SETTING POWDER.

INSTRUCTIONS: BEGIN BY APPLYING A PRIMER TO CREATE A SMOOTH BASE AND HELP THE MAKEUP ADHERE BETTER. COVER THE ENTIRE FACE WITH GREEN FACE PAINT, ENSURING EVEN COVERAGE FOR A STRIKING WITCHY COMPLEXION. SET THE PAINT WITH TRANSLUCENT POWDER TO KEEP THE MAKEUP IN PLACE AND PREVENT IT FROM SMUDGING.

EYES:

TOOLS: BLACK EYESHADOW, EYELINER, GREEN CONTACT LENSES, MASCARA.

INSTRUCTIONS: APPLY BLACK EYESHADOW TO THE EYELIDS, BLENDING IT OUTWARD TO CREATE A SMOKY, SINISTER LOOK. USE EYELINER TO DEFINE THE EYES, ACCENTUATING THE SHAPE WITH A DRAMATIC WING. ENHANCE THE EFFECT WITH GREEN CONTACT LENSES TO GIVE THE EYES AN EERIE, MAGICAL GLOW. FINISH WITH MASCARA TO ADD VOLUME AND DEFINITION TO THE LASHES.

FACE DETAILING:

TOOLS: BLACK FACE PAINT, FINE BRUSH, BLACK FOREHEAD ORNAMENT (E.G., SPIDER DESIGN).

INSTRUCTIONS: USE BLACK FACE PAINT TO DRAW INTRICATE, WEB-LIKE DESIGNS AROUND THE EYES, EXTENDING OUTWARD FROM THE CORNERS. PLACE A BLACK SPIDER OR SIMILAR ORNAMENT IN THE CENTER OF THE FOREHEAD TO ADD AN EXTRA TOUCH OF WICKEDNESS. ENSURE THAT THE DESIGNS ARE SYMMETRICAL AND CLEANLY DRAWN TO CREATE A POLISHED LOOK.

LIPS:

TOOLS: BLACK LIPSTICK, LIP LINER.

INSTRUCTIONS: OUTLINE THE LIPS WITH BLACK LIP LINER TO DEFINE THEIR SHAPE, THEN FILL IN WITH BLACK LIPSTICK. THE DARK LIPS SHOULD COMPLEMENT THE OVERALL GREEN AND BLACK COLOR SCHEME, ADDING TO THE WICKED APPEARANCE OF THE WITCH.

HAIR & ACCESSORIES:

TOOLS: BLACK WIG OR HAIR DYE, GREEN AND BLACK EARRINGS, HAIR GEL.

INSTRUCTIONS: STYLE THE HAIR INTO A SLEEK, POLISHED LOOK USING A BLACK WIG OR HAIR DYE IF NECESSARY. USE HAIR GEL TO SMOOTH ANY FLYAWAYS AND MAINTAIN THE SLEEK APPEARANCE. ADD GREEN AND BLACK EARRINGS TO COMPLEMENT THE MAKEUP AND COSTUME, ENHANCING THE OVERALL WITCHY VIBE.

COSTUME:

TOOLS: WITCH COSTUME WITH GOTHIC ELEMENTS, GREEN AND BLACK ACCENTS, RED JEWEL NECKLACE.

INSTRUCTIONS: WEAR A WITCH COSTUME THAT INCORPORATES GOTHIC ELEMENTS LIKE LACE OR HIGH COLLARS, WITH GREEN AND BLACK ACCENTS TO MATCH THE MAKEUP. ADD A RED JEWEL NECKLACE FOR A STRIKING CONTRAST, DRAWING ATTENTION TO THE CENTER OF THE CHEST. THE COSTUME SHOULD BE ELEGANT YET SINISTER, REFLECTING THE MALEVOLENT CHARACTER OF THE WITCH.

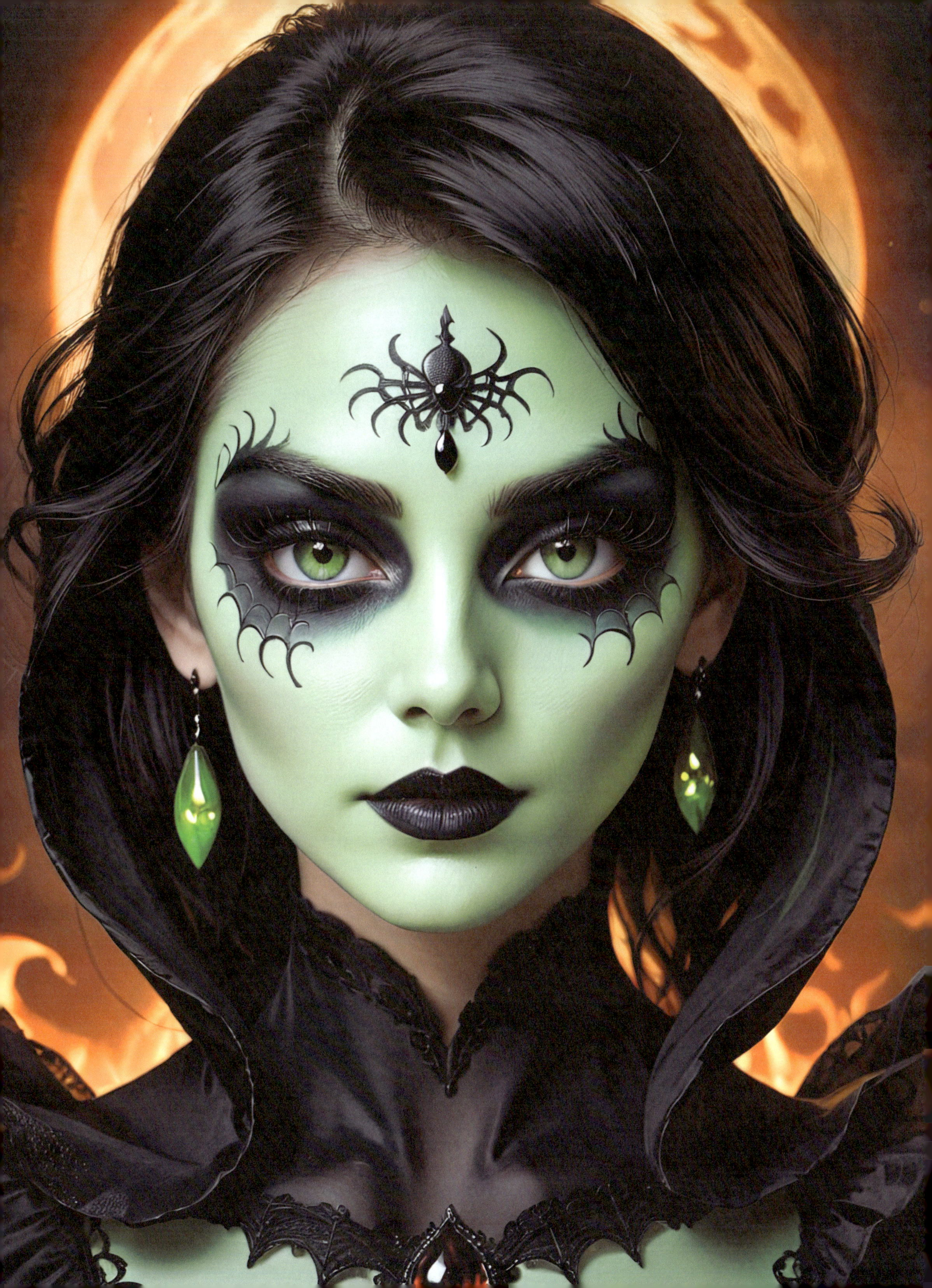

"GOTHIC HALLOWEEN"

STEP-BY-STEP INSTRUCTIONS:

SKIN PREPARATION:

TOOLS: PRIMER, WHITE FACE PAINT, TRANSLUCENT SETTING POWDER.

INSTRUCTIONS: BEGIN BY APPLYING A PRIMER TO CREATE A SMOOTH SURFACE AND TO HELP THE MAKEUP ADHERE BETTER. COVER THE ENTIRE FACE WITH WHITE FACE PAINT, ENSURING AN EVEN AND SMOOTH BASE. SET THE FACE PAINT WITH A TRANSLUCENT SETTING POWDER TO LOCK IN THE MAKEUP AND PREVENT SMUDGING.

EYES:

TOOLS: BLACK EYESHADOW, EYELINER, GREEN CONTACT LENSES, MASCARA.

INSTRUCTIONS: APPLY BLACK EYESHADOW AROUND THE EYES, EXTENDING IT OUTWARD AND UPWARD TO CREATE A SMOKY, DRAMATIC EFFECT. USE EYELINER TO OUTLINE THE EYES, EMPHASIZING THE UPPER AND LOWER LASH LINES. APPLY GREEN CONTACT LENSES TO GIVE THE EYES A HAUNTING, OTHERWORLDLY GLOW. FINISH WITH MASCARA TO ADD VOLUME AND DEFINITION TO THE LASHES.

FACE DETAILING:

TOOLS: BLACK FACE PAINT, FINE BRUSH, BLACK FOREHEAD JEWEL, AND SPIDER WEB STENCILS.

INSTRUCTIONS: USING BLACK FACE PAINT AND A FINE BRUSH, CREATE INTRICATE DESIGNS ACROSS THE FOREHEAD AND AROUND THE EYES, FOCUSING ON A SPIDER WEB PATTERN. START FROM THE CENTER OF THE FOREHEAD AND EXTEND THE WEB OUTWARD, ENSURING SYMMETRY. ADD A BLACK JEWEL OR ORNAMENT IN THE MIDDLE OF THE FOREHEAD FOR A GOTHIC TOUCH. USE STENCILS IF NEEDED TO ENSURE PRECISION IN THE WEB DESIGN.

NOSE AND LIPS:

TOOLS: BLACK FACE PAINT, BLACK LIPSTICK, FINE BRUSH.

INSTRUCTIONS: PAINT THE TIP OF THE NOSE BLACK, MIMICKING A SKULL'S NOSE CAVITY FOR A SKELETAL EFFECT. FOR THE LIPS, APPLY BLACK LIPSTICK, KEEPING THE EDGES SHARP. TO ADD A STITCHED EFFECT, USE A FINE BRUSH TO DRAW THIN, HORIZONTAL LINES EXTENDING FROM THE CORNERS OF THE MOUTH OUTWARD.

HAIR & ACCESSORIES:

TOOLS: HAIRPINS, BLACK HAIR DYE OR WIG, ORANGE AND BLACK EARRINGS, HAIR GEL.

INSTRUCTIONS: STYLE THE HAIR INTO NEAT BUNS ON EITHER SIDE OF THE HEAD USING HAIRPINS. IF NEEDED, USE BLACK HAIR DYE OR A WIG TO ACHIEVE A DEEP, DARK TONE. ADD HAIR GEL TO KEEP THE STYLE IN PLACE AND ENSURE A SLEEK LOOK. CHOOSE ORANGE AND BLACK EARRINGS TO COMPLEMENT THE HALLOWEEN THEME, ADDING A POP OF COLOR AGAINST THE DARK COSTUME.

COSTUME:

TOOLS: GOTHIC DRESS WITH LACE DETAILS, BLACK AND ORANGE ACCESSORIES, PUMPKIN PENDANT NECKLACE.

INSTRUCTIONS: WEAR A GOTHICSTYLE DRESS, PREFERABLY WITH LACE DETAILS AND A HIGH COLLAR, TO ENHANCE THE HALLOWEEN LOOK. ADD BLACK AND ORANGE ACCESSORIES TO TIE IN WITH THE MAKEUP AND OVERALL THEME. FINISH THE OUTFIT WITH A STATEMENT PUMPKIN PENDANT NECKLACE TO EMPHASIZE THE HALLOWEEN SPIRIT, DRAWING ATTENTION TO THE CHEST AREA.

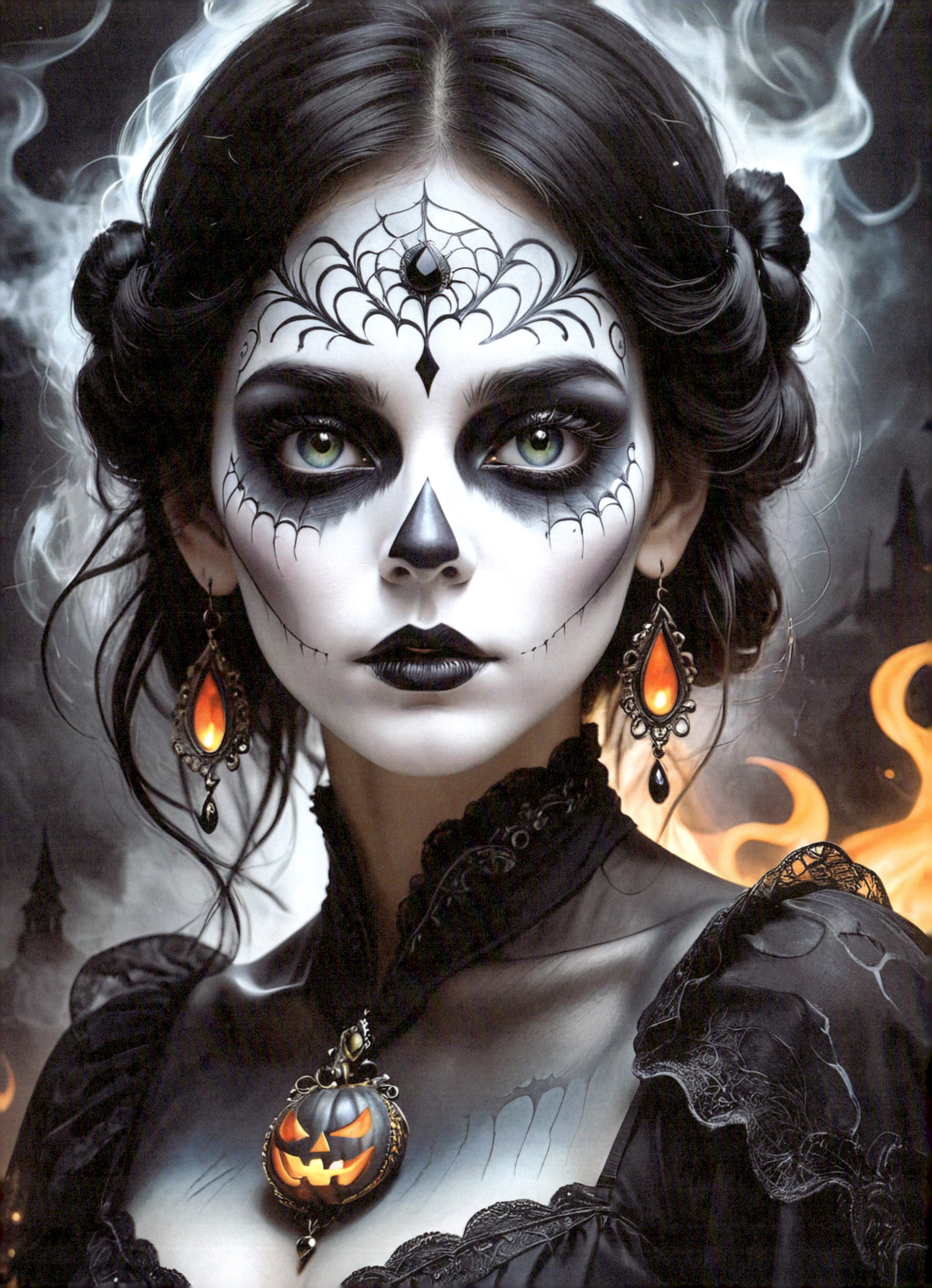

"ICY ENCHANTRESS"

STEP-BY-STEP INSTRUCTIONS:

SKIN PREPARATION:

TOOLS: PRIMER, LIGHT BLUE FACE PAINT, TRANSLUCENT SETTING POWDER.

INSTRUCTIONS: BEGIN BY APPLYING A PRIMER TO CREATE A SMOOTH BASE FOR THE MAKEUP. COVER THE ENTIRE FACE WITH LIGHT BLUE FACE PAINT, BLENDING EVENLY TO ACHIEVE A COOL, ICY COMPLEXION. SET THE PAINT WITH TRANSLUCENT POWDER TO PREVENT ANY SMUDGING AND TO KEEP THE MAKEUP LONG-LASTING.

EYES:

TOOLS: DARK BLUE AND BLACK EYESHADOW, EYELINER, ICY BLUE CONTACT LENSES, MASCARA.

INSTRUCTIONS: APPLY DARK BLUE EYESHADOW AROUND THE EYES, EXTENDING IT OUTWARD TO CREATE A DRAMATIC, FROSTY LOOK. BLEND BLACK EYESHADOW INTO THE OUTER CORNERS TO ADD DEPTH AND INTENSITY. USE EYELINER TO OUTLINE THE EYES, FOCUSING ON CREATING A SHARP, DEFINED WING. ADD ICY BLUE CONTACT LENSES FOR A PIERCING, ENCHANTING GAZE. FINISH WITH MASCARA TO DEFINE THE LASHES AND ENHANCE THE OVERALL EYE MAKEUP.

FACE DETAILING:

TOOLS: BLACK FACE PAINT, FINE BRUSH.

INSTRUCTIONS: USE BLACK FACE PAINT TO CREATE INTRICATE DESIGNS ON THE FOREHEAD, RESEMBLING FROZEN FLAMES OR SHARP, ICY PATTERNS. DRAW THE DESIGNS SYMMETRICALLY, EXTENDING THEM FROM THE CENTER OF THE FOREHEAD AND AROUND THE EYES. ADD SUBTLE SHADING WITHIN THE DESIGNS TO CREATE DEPTH AND A MORE DYNAMIC, THREE-DIMENSIONAL EFFECT.

LIPS:

TOOLS: DARK BLUE LIPSTICK, LIP LINER.

INSTRUCTIONS: OUTLINE THE LIPS WITH A DARK BLUE LIP LINER TO DEFINE THEIR SHAPE, THEN FILL IN WITH DARK BLUE LIPSTICK. THE LIPS SHOULD APPEAR BOLD AND MATCH THE COOL, ICY THEME OF THE OVERALL LOOK, ADDING A TOUCH OF WINTERY ELEGANCE.

HAIR & ACCESSORIES:

TOOLS: BLUE WIG OR HAIR DYE, GOLD HOOP EARRINGS, HAIR GEL.

INSTRUCTIONS: STYLE THE HAIR INTO LOOSE, VOLUMINOUS WAVES USING A BLUE WIG OR HAIR DYE IF NECESSARY. USE HAIR GEL TO MAINTAIN THE WAVES AND KEEP THEM IN PLACE. ADD LARGE GOLD HOOP EARRINGS TO PROVIDE A STRIKING CONTRAST AGAINST THE BLUE TONES OF THE MAKEUP AND HAIR, ENHANCING THE REGAL APPEARANCE OF THE ENCHANTRESS.

COSTUME:

TOOLS: BLACK AND BLUE GOWN WITH ICY DETAILS, GOLD ACCENTS.

INSTRUCTIONS: WEAR A GOWN IN BLACK AND BLUE TONES, PREFERABLY WITH ICY OR FROST-LIKE DETAILS TO COMPLEMENT THE MAKEUP. INCORPORATE GOLD ACCENTS, SUCH AS JEWELRY OR EMBROIDERY, TO ADD AN ELEGANT TOUCH. THE COSTUME SHOULD REFLECT THE ICY, MYSTICAL NATURE OF THE CHARACTER, WITH A BLEND OF COLD AND REGAL ELEMENTS.

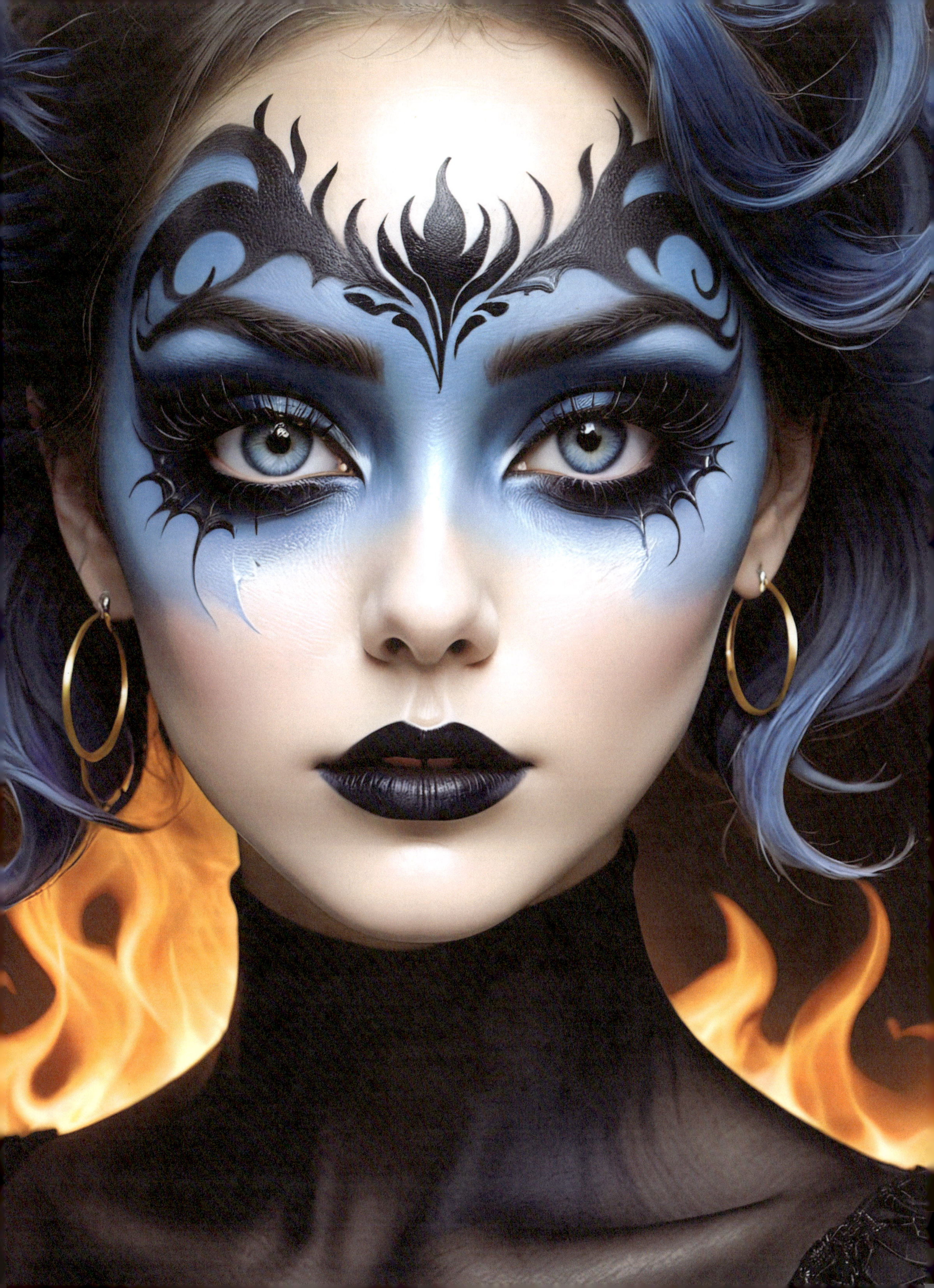

"MYSTICAL SKULL"

STEP-BY-STEP INSTRUCTIONS:

SKIN PREPARATION:

TOOLS: PRIMER, WHITE FACE PAINT, TRANSLUCENT SETTING POWDER.

INSTRUCTIONS: BEGIN BY APPLYING A PRIMER TO CREATE A SMOOTH, EVEN BASE. APPLY WHITE FACE PAINT OVER THE ENTIRE FACE, ENSURING EVEN COVERAGE TO CREATE A GHOSTLY, SKELETAL COMPLEXION. SET THE FACE PAINT WITH A TRANSLUCENT SETTING POWDER TO LOCK IT IN AND PREVENT SMUDGING.

EYES:

TOOLS: BLACK EYESHADOW, EYELINER, GREEN CONTACT LENSES, MASCARA.

INSTRUCTIONS: APPLY BLACK EYESHADOW AROUND THE EYES, EXTENDING IT OUTWARD TO CREATE A HOLLOW, SUNKEN APPEARANCE. BLEND THE EDGES CAREFULLY FOR A SMOOTH TRANSITION INTO THE WHITE BASE. USE EYELINER TO INTENSIFY THE LOOK BY DEFINING THE UPPER AND LOWER LASH LINES. ADD GREEN CONTACT LENSES TO GIVE THE EYES AN EERIE, HAUNTING GLOW. FINISH WITH MASCARA TO DEFINE THE LASHES AND ENHANCE THE DEPTH OF THE EYES.

FACE DETAILING:

TOOLS: BLACK FACE PAINT, FINE BRUSH, BLACK FOREHEAD JEWEL.

INSTRUCTIONS: USING BLACK FACE PAINT AND A FINE BRUSH, CREATE INTRICATE DESIGNS ON THE FOREHEAD, FOCUSING ON A CENTRAL, SYMMETRICAL PATTERN. DRAW ADDITIONAL DESIGNS AROUND THE EYES, RESEMBLING CRACKED OR WEB-LIKE STRUCTURES THAT ENHANCE THE SKELETAL APPEARANCE. PLACE A BLACK JEWEL OR ORNAMENT AT THE CENTER OF THE FOREHEAD TO ADD A MYSTICAL TOUCH. CONTINUE THE DESIGN BY DRAWING A STITCHED EFFECT AROUND THE MOUTH, EXTENDING FROM THE CORNERS OF THE LIPS TO MIMIC A SEWN-SHUT LOOK.

LIPS:

TOOLS: BLACK LIPSTICK, FINE BRUSH.

INSTRUCTIONS: APPLY BLACK LIPSTICK TO THE LIPS, KEEPING THE EDGES SHARP AND PRECISE. TO COMPLEMENT THE STITCHED DESIGN, USE A FINE BRUSH TO EXTEND THE BLACK LINES FROM THE CORNERS OF THE MOUTH, ENHANCING THE ILLUSION OF A SEWN, SKELETAL GRIN.

HAIR & ACCESSORIES:

TOOLS: HAIRPINS, BLACK HAIR DYE OR WIG, RED GEMSTONE EARRINGS, HAIR GEL.

INSTRUCTIONS: STYLE THE HAIR INTO LOOSE WAVES OR CURLS, USING HAIRPINS TO HOLD ANY INTRICATE STYLES IN PLACE. IF NEEDED, USE BLACK HAIR DYE OR A WIG TO ACHIEVE A DEEP, DARK TONE. ADD HAIR GEL TO KEEP THE STYLE SMOOTH AND NEAT. COMPLEMENT THE LOOK WITH RED GEMSTONE EARRINGS TO ADD A TOUCH OF COLOR THAT CONTRASTS WITH THE BLACK AND WHITE MAKEUP, GIVING THE LOOK AN ELEGANT, GOTHIC FINISH.

COSTUME:

TOOLS: GOTHIC LACE DRESS, RED GEMSTONE NECKLACE, BLACK LACE GLOVES.

INSTRUCTIONS: WEAR A GOTHIC LACE DRESS WITH INTRICATE PATTERNS THAT COMPLEMENT THE DETAILED FACE DESIGNS. ADD A RED GEMSTONE NECKLACE TO TIE IN WITH THE EARRINGS, CREATING A FOCAL POINT ON THE CHEST. COMPLETE THE OUTFIT WITH BLACK LACE GLOVES TO ENHANCE THE GOTHIC, SKELETAL THEME AND ADD A TOUCH OF SOPHISTICATION TO THE OVERALL LOOK.

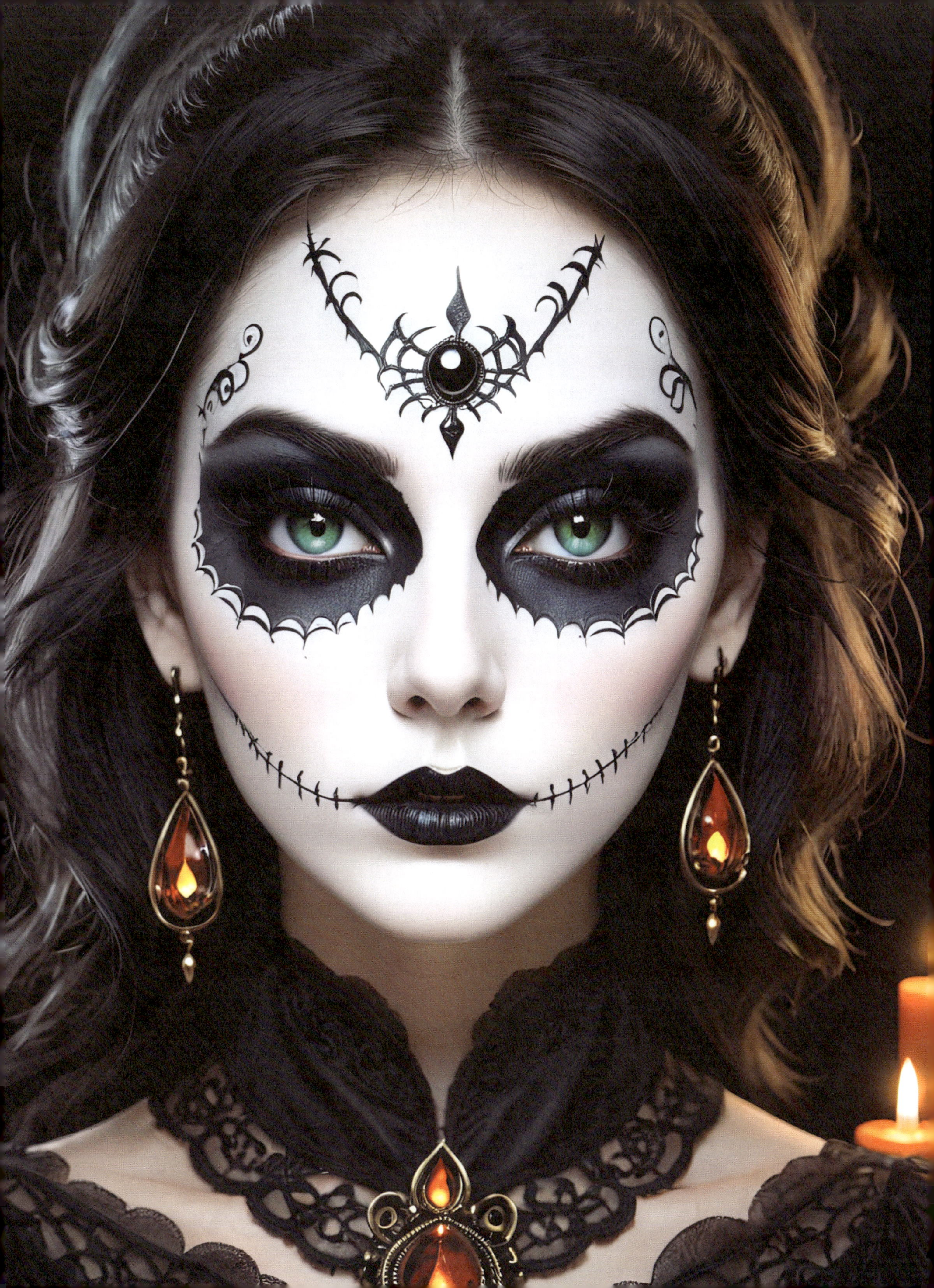

"EMERALD ENIGMA"

STEP-BY-STEP INSTRUCTIONS:

SKIN PREPARATION:

TOOLS: PRIMER, LIGHT FOUNDATION, TRANSLUCENT SETTING POWDER.

INSTRUCTIONS: BEGIN BY APPLYING A PRIMER TO CREATE A SMOOTH, EVEN BASE. USE A LIGHT FOUNDATION TO EVEN OUT THE SKIN TONE, ENSURING A FLAWLESS COMPLEXION. SET THE FOUNDATION WITH A TRANSLUCENT POWDER TO KEEP IT IN PLACE AND PROVIDE A MATTE FINISH.

EYES:

TOOLS: DARK GREEN AND BLACK EYESHADOW, EYELINER, GREEN CONTACT LENSES, MASCARA.

INSTRUCTIONS: APPLY DARK GREEN EYESHADOW AROUND THE EYES, BLENDING IT OUTWARD AND INTO THE CREASE TO CREATE A SMOKY, MYSTERIOUS EFFECT. ADD BLACK EYESHADOW TO THE OUTER CORNERS TO INTENSIFY THE LOOK AND CREATE DEPTH. USE EYELINER TO DEFINE THE EYES, DRAWING A SHARP LINE ALONG THE UPPER AND LOWER LASH LINES. APPLY GREEN CONTACT LENSES TO GIVE THE EYES A STRIKING, OTHERWORLDLY APPEARANCE. FINISH WITH MASCARA TO ENHANCE THE LASHES AND COMPLETE THE DRAMATIC EYE MAKEUP.

FACE DETAILING:

TOOLS: BLACK FACE PAINT, FINE BRUSH, BLACK FOREHEAD JEWEL.

INSTRUCTIONS: USING BLACK FACE PAINT AND A FINE BRUSH, CREATE INTRICATE DESIGNS ON THE FOREHEAD, FOCUSING ON A CENTRAL SYMMETRICAL PATTERN, PERHAPS RESEMBLING A SPIDER OR OTHER MYSTICAL SYMBOL. EXTEND THE DESIGN AROUND THE EYES WITH ADDITIONAL PATTERNS THAT ENHANCE THE GOTHIC, EERIE AESTHETIC. PLACE A BLACK JEWEL AT THE CENTER OF THE FOREHEAD TO SERVE AS A FOCAL POINT AND ADD AN ELEMENT OF MYSTIQUE.

LIPS:

TOOLS: BLACK LIPSTICK, LIP LINER.

INSTRUCTIONS: OUTLINE THE LIPS WITH A BLACK LIP LINER TO CREATE A DEFINED SHAPE. FILL IN THE LIPS WITH BLACK LIPSTICK FOR A BOLD, DRAMATIC CONTRAST AGAINST THE LIGHTER SKIN. THE DARK LIPS SHOULD COMPLEMENT THE INTENSE EYE MAKEUP, CONTRIBUTING TO THE OVERALL GOTHIC THEME.

HAIR & ACCESSORIES:

TOOLS: HAIRPINS, BLACK AND GREEN HAIR DYE OR WIG, BLACK GEMSTONE EARRINGS, HAIR GEL.

INSTRUCTIONS: STYLE THE HAIR INTO ELEGANT, VOLUMINOUS CURLS OR WAVES, USING HAIRPINS TO HOLD THE STYLE IN PLACE. IF NECESSARY, USE BLACK AND GREEN HAIR DYE OR A WIG TO ACHIEVE THE DESIRED LOOK. USE HAIR GEL TO SMOOTH ANY FLYAWAYS AND MAINTAIN THE HAIRSTYLE. ADD BLACK GEMSTONE EARRINGS TO MATCH THE JEWEL ON THE FOREHEAD, ENHANCING THE OVERALL GOTHIC, MYSTICAL APPEARANCE.

COSTUME:

TOOLS: BLACK LACE DRESS WITH GOTHIC ELEMENTS, EMERALD AND BLACK JEWELRY, SHEER SHAWL.

INSTRUCTIONS: WEAR A BLACK LACE DRESS WITH INTRICATE GOTHIC DETAILS THAT COMPLEMENT THE DARK, MYSTERIOUS MAKEUP. ADD EMERALD AND BLACK JEWELRY, SUCH AS A PENDANT OR BROOCH, TO TIE IN WITH THE EMERALD TONES IN THE MAKEUP. CONSIDER ADDING A SHEER SHAWL OR CAPE TO THE ENSEMBLE TO CREATE A MORE ETHEREAL, FLOWING SILHOUETTE THAT MATCHES THE ENIGMA OF THE CHARACTER.

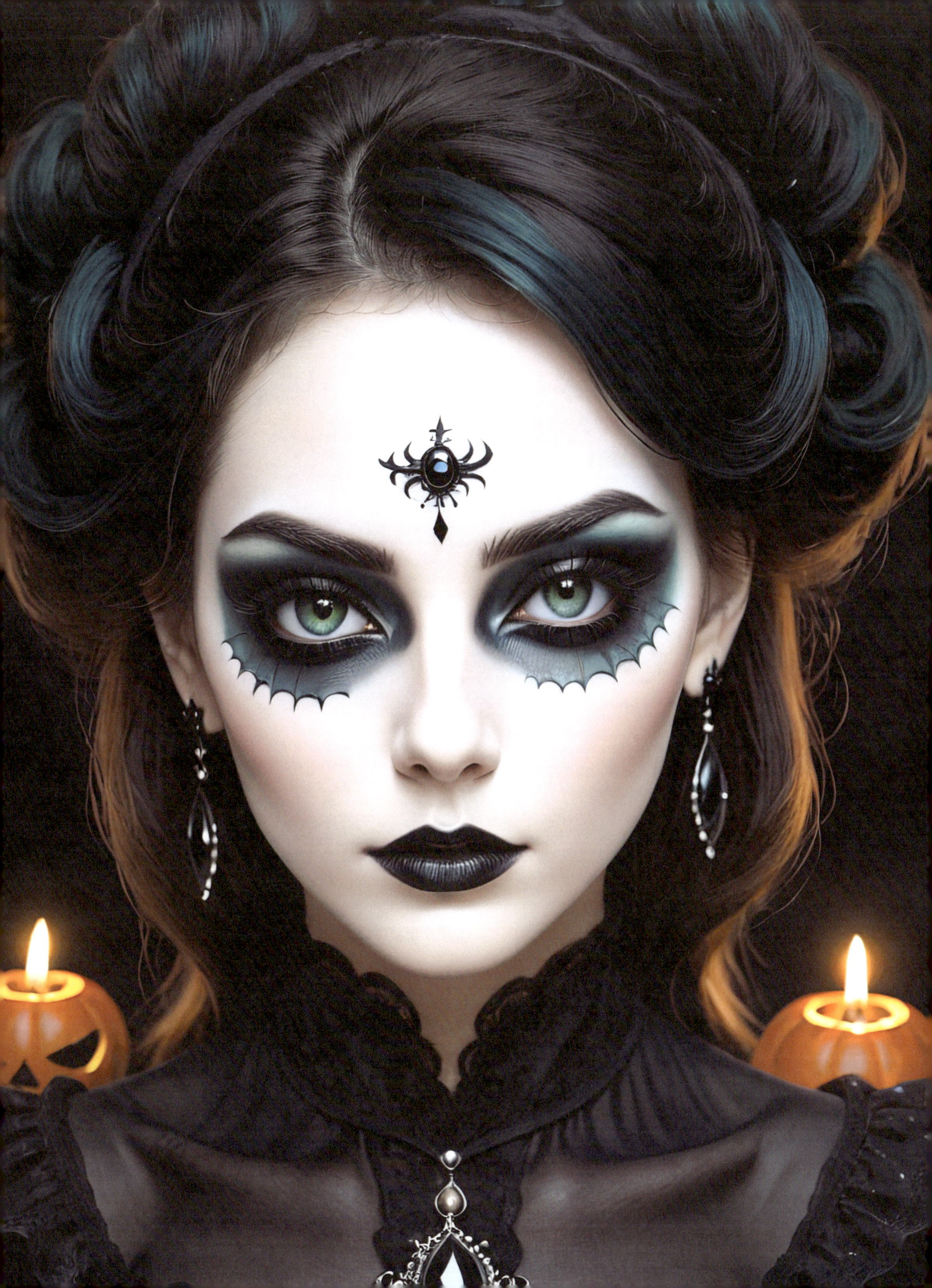

"BLACK HALLOWEEN COVER LOOK"

STEP-BY-STEP INSTRUCTIONS:

THIS IS THE MAKEUP INSTRUCTION FOR THE LOOK FEATURED ON THE COVER OF "BLACK HALLOWEEN."

SKIN PREPARATION:

TOOLS: PRIMER, WHITE FACE PAINT, TRANSLUCENT SETTING POWDER.

INSTRUCTIONS: START BY APPLYING A PRIMER TO ENSURE THE MAKEUP LASTS LONGER AND GOES ON SMOOTHLY. COVER THE ENTIRE FACE WITH WHITE FACE PAINT, BLENDING EVENLY TO CREATE A GHOSTLY, SKELETAL BASE. SET THE FACE PAINT WITH TRANSLUCENT POWDER TO KEEP IT IN PLACE AND PREVENT SMUDGING.

EYES:

TOOLS: BLACK EYESHADOW, EYELINER, GREEN CONTACT LENSES, MASCARA.

INSTRUCTIONS: APPLY BLACK EYESHADOW AROUND THE EYES, EXTENDING IT OUTWARD TO CREATE A HOLLOW, SUNKEN LOOK. BLEND THE EDGES CAREFULLY INTO THE WHITE BASE TO ACHIEVE A SMOOTH TRANSITION. USE BLACK EYELINER TO INTENSIFY THE EFFECT BY DEFINING THE UPPER AND LOWER LASH LINES. ADD GREEN CONTACT LENSES FOR A HAUNTING, PIERCING GAZE. FINISH WITH MASCARA TO DEFINE AND ENHANCE THE LASHES, COMPLETING THE EERIE EYE LOOK.

FACE DETAILING:

TOOLS: BLACK FACE PAINT, FINE BRUSH.

INSTRUCTIONS: USING BLACK FACE PAINT AND A FINE BRUSH, DRAW THE SKELETAL FEATURES, FOCUSING ON THE NOSE AND MOUTH AREAS. CREATE A SKELETAL NOSE BY FILLING IN THE TIP OF THE NOSE WITH BLACK PAINT. FOR THE MOUTH, DRAW A SERIES OF VERTICAL LINES EXTENDING FROM THE CORNERS, MIMICKING THE LOOK OF A STITCHED OR CRACKED JAW. ADD ADDITIONAL SKELETAL DETAILS AROUND THE FOREHEAD AND CHEEKS, ENSURING THE LINES ARE SHARP AND SYMMETRICAL FOR A POLISHED, HAUNTING EFFECT.

LIPS:

TOOLS: BLACK LIPSTICK, FINE BRUSH.

INSTRUCTIONS: OUTLINE THE LIPS WITH BLACK LIP LINER, THEN FILL IN WITH BLACK LIPSTICK FOR A BOLD, STRIKING LOOK. USE A FINE BRUSH TO EXTEND THE BLACK LINES FROM THE CORNERS OF THE MOUTH, INTEGRATING THEM INTO THE SKELETAL DESIGN FOR A COHESIVE LOOK.

HAIR & ACCESSORIES:

TOOLS: HAIRPINS, BLACK HAIR DYE OR WIG, HAIR GEL.

INSTRUCTIONS: STYLE THE HAIR INTO NEAT, VOLUMINOUS BUNS ON EITHER SIDE OF THE HEAD, SECURING THEM WITH HAIRPINS. IF NECESSARY, USE BLACK HAIR DYE OR A WIG TO ACHIEVE THE DESIRED DARK, GOTHIC LOOK. APPLY HAIR GEL TO SMOOTH ANY FLYAWAYS AND KEEP THE HAIRSTYLE SLEEK AND POLISHED.

COSTUME:

TOOLS: BLACK LACE DRESS WITH GOTHIC ELEMENTS.

INSTRUCTIONS: WEAR A BLACK LACE DRESS WITH GOTHIC DETAILS, SUCH AS HIGH COLLARS AND INTRICATE LACE PATTERNS, TO COMPLEMENT THE SKELETAL MAKEUP. THE COSTUME SHOULD ENHANCE THE EERIE, GHOSTLY ATMOSPHERE OF THE COVER IMAGE, COMPLETING THE "BLACK HALLOWEEN"

THANK YOU FOR CHOOSING OUR BOOK AND FOR DIVING INTO THE WORLD OF HALLOWEEN MAKEUP.

WE HOPE THAT OUR INSTRUCTIONS, INSPIRATIONS, AND TIPS HAVE HELPED YOU CREATE UNFORGETTABLE LOOKS THAT ADDED MAGIC AND THRILLS TO YOUR HALLOWEEN CELEBRATIONS. EACH PROJECT IN THIS BOOK WAS CRAFTED WITH YOU IN MIND — YOUR CREATIVITY, YOUR PASSION, AND YOUR DESIRE TO EXPLORE NEW AND EXCITING WAYS TO EXPRESS YOURSELF.

REMEMBER, MAKEUP IS AN ART FORM WITHOUT LIMITS. EVERY BRUSHSTROKE, EVERY DETAIL IS AN OPPORTUNITY TO CREATE SOMETHING UNIQUE THAT REFLECTS YOUR PERSONALITY AND IMAGINATION. LET THIS BOOK BE AN INSPIRATION FOR YOU FOR YEARS TO COME, ENCOURAGING FURTHER EXPERIMENTATION AND DISCOVERY OF NEW TECHNIQUES.

ONCE AGAIN, THANK YOU FOR PURCHASING OUR BOOK. YOUR SUPPORT ALLOWS US TO CONTINUE CREATING MATERIALS THAT HELP YOU GROW AND ENJOY THE ART OF MAKEUP. WE WISH YOU MANY JOYFUL AND CREATIVE MOMENTS WITH MAKEUP, AND MANY SCARY AND UNFORGETTABLE HALLOWEENS!